CONTENTS

Preface 4

Acknowledgements 5

Executive summary 6

BACKGROUND 10

PART 1: GLOBAL BURDEN OF DIABETES 20
1.1 Mortality from high blood glucose, including diabetes 21
1.2 Prevalence of diabetes and associated risk factors 25
1.3 Burden and trends in the complications of diabetes 30
1.4 Summary 31

PART 2: PREVENTING DIABETES 34
2.1 Population-based prevention 35
2.2 Preventing diabetes in people at high risk 40
2.3 Summary 42

PART 3: MANAGING DIABETES 46
3.1 Diagnosis and early detection 47
3.2 Management of diabetes – core components 49
3.3 Integrated management of diabetes and other chronic health conditions 54
3.4 Access to essential medicines and basic technologies 58
3.5 Summary 61

PART 4. NATIONAL CAPACITY FOR PREVENTION AND CONTROL OF DIABETES: A SNAPSHOT 66
4.1 National policies and plans for diabetes 68
4.2 National guidelines and protocols 69
4.3 Availability of essential medicines and technologies 71
4.4 Surveillance and monitoring 74
4.5 Summary 74

CONCLUSIONS AND RECOMMENDATIONS 76

ANNEXES 82
Annex A. Current WHO recommendations for the diagnostic criteria for diabetes and intermediate hyperglycaemia 83
Annex B. Methods for estimating diabetes prevalence, overweight and obesity prevalence, mortality attributable to high blood glucose, and price of insulin 84

PREFACE

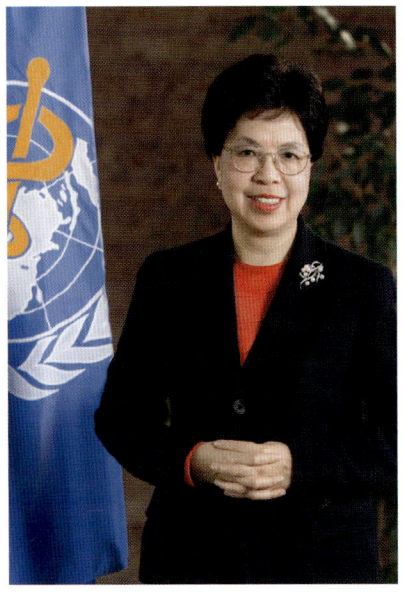

Diabetes is on the rise. No longer a disease of predominantly rich nations, the prevalence of diabetes is steadily increasing everywhere, most markedly in the world's middle-income countries.

Unfortunately, in many settings the lack of effective policies to create supportive environments for healthy lifestyles and the lack of access to quality health care means that the prevention and treatment of diabetes, particularly for people of modest means, are not being pursued.

When diabetes is uncontrolled, it has dire consequences for health and well-being.

In addition, diabetes and its complications impact harshly on the finances of individuals and their families, and the economies of nations. People with diabetes who depend on life-saving insulin pay the ultimate price when access to affordable insulin is lacking.

In an effort to address this growing health challenge, since early this decade world leaders have committed to reducing the burden of diabetes as one of four priority noncommunicable diseases (NCDs).

As part of the 2030 Agenda for Sustainable Development, Member States have set an ambitious target to reduce premature mortality from NCDs – including diabetes – by one third; achieve universal health coverage; and provide access to affordable essential medicines – all by 2030.

We have an enormous task at hand, which is why I welcome this first WHO *Global report on diabetes*. The report makes an important contribution to our understanding of diabetes and its consequences.

It advances our understanding of trends in diabetes prevalence, of the contribution of high blood glucose (including diabetes) to premature mortality, and of what action governments are taking to prevent and control diabetes.

From the analysis it is clear we need stronger responses not only from different sectors of government, but also from civil society and people with diabetes themselves, and also producers of food and manufacturers of medicines and medical technologies.

The report reminds us that effectively addressing diabetes does not just happen: it is the result of collective consensus and public investment in interventions that are affordable, cost-effective and based on the best available science.

Please join me in ensuring that the findings of this report are used and its recommendations implemented so that we may indeed halt the rise in diabetes.

Dr Margaret Chan
Director-General
WHO

ACKNOWLEDGEMENTS

This report benefited from the dedication, support and expertise of a number of WHO staff and external collaborators.

Staff from WHO headquarters: Gojka Roglic coordinated and produced the report in collaboration with an editorial team comprising Cherian Varghese, Leanne Riley and Alison Harvey. Etienne Krug and Ala Alwan provided strategic direction. Statistical analysis was provided by Melanie Cowan and Stefan Savin. Timothy Armstrong, Nicholas Banatvala, Douglas Bettcher, Francesco Branca, Edouard Tursan d'Espaignet, Suzanne Hill, Ivo Kocur, Cécile Macé, Silvio Mariotti, Colin Mathers, Leendert Nederveen, Chizuru Nishida, Laura Sminkey, Gretchen Stevens, Meindert Van Hilten, Temo Waqanivalu and Stephen Whiting provided technical input. The country profiles (available online) were prepared by Melanie Cowan with assistance from Nisreen Abdel Latif, Maggie Awadalla, Sebastian Brown, Alison Commar, Karna Dhiravani, Jessica Sing Sum Ho, Kacem Iaych, Andre Ilbawi, Xin Ya Lim, Leanne Riley, Slim Slama and Juana Willumsen. Elena Altieri provided communications support. Joel Tarel, Hélène Dufays and Melissa Foxman Burns provided administrative support.

Staff from WHO regional offices: Alberto Barcelo, Padmini Angela De Silva, Gampo Dorji, Jill Farrington, Gauden Galea, Anselm Hennis, Warrick Junsuk Kim, Hai-Rim Shin, Steven Shongwe, Slim Slama, and Thaksaphon Thamarangasi reviewed the draft report and provided technical input.

WHO wishes to thank the following external contributors and reviewers whose expertise made this report possible:

Stephen Colagiuri, Pamela Donggo, Edward Gregg, Viswanathan Mohan, Nigel Unwin, Rhys Williams and John Yudkin for providing guidance on content.

James Bentham, Goodarz Danaei, Mariachiara Di Cesare, Majid Ezzati, Kaveh Hajifathalian, Vasilis Kontis, Yuan Lu and Bin Zhou for data analyses and estimates.

David Beran, Stephen Colagiuri, Edward Gregg, Viswanathan Mohan, Ambady Ramachandran, Jeffrey Stephens, David Stuckler, John Yudkin, Nicholas Wareham, Rhys Williams and Ping Zhang for writing sections of the report.

Peter Bennett, Pascal Bovet, David Cavan, Michael Engelgau, Ayesha Motala, Simon O'Neill, Eugene Sobngwi, Nikhil Tandon and Jaakko Tuomilehto for peer review.

Angela Burton for technical editing.

EXECUTIVE SUMMARY

Diabetes is a serious, chronic disease that occurs either when the pancreas does not produce enough insulin (a hormone that regulates blood sugar, or glucose), or when the body cannot effectively use the insulin it produces. Diabetes is an important public health problem, one of four priority noncommunicable diseases (NCDs) targeted for action by world leaders. Both the number of cases and the prevalence of diabetes have been steadily increasing over the past few decades.

GLOBAL BURDEN

Globally, an estimated 422 million adults were living with diabetes in 2014, compared to 108 million in 1980. The global prevalence (age-standardized) of diabetes has nearly doubled since 1980, rising from 4.7% to 8.5% in the adult population. This reflects an increase in associated risk factors such as being overweight or obese. Over the past decade, diabetes prevalence has risen faster in low- and middle-income countries than in high-income countries.

Diabetes caused 1.5 million deaths in 2012. Higher-than-optimal blood glucose caused an additional 2.2 million deaths, by increasing the risks of cardiovascular and other diseases. Forty-three percent of these 3.7 million deaths occur before the age of 70 years. The percentage of deaths attributable to high blood glucose or diabetes that occurs prior to age 70 is higher in low- and middle-income countries than in high-income countries.

Because sophisticated laboratory tests are usually required to distinguish between type 1 diabetes (which requires insulin injections for survival) and type 2 diabetes (where the body cannot properly use the insulin it produces), separate global estimates of diabetes prevalence for type 1 and type 2 do not exist. The majority of people with diabetes are affected by type 2 diabetes. This used to occur nearly entirely among adults, but now occurs in children too.

COMPLICATIONS

Diabetes of all types can lead to complications in many parts of the body and can increase the overall risk of dying prematurely. Possible complications include heart attack, stroke, kidney failure, leg amputation, vision loss and nerve damage. In pregnancy, poorly controlled diabetes increases the risk of fetal death and other complications.

ECONOMIC IMPACT

Diabetes and its complications bring about substantial economic loss to people with diabetes and their families, and to health systems and national economies through direct medical costs and loss of work and wages. While the major cost drivers are hospital and outpatient care, a contributing factor is the rise in cost for analogue insulins[1] which are increasingly prescribed despite little evidence that they provide significant advantages over cheaper human insulins.

---

1. These are insulins derived from human insulin by modifying its structure to change the pharmacokinetic profile.

PREVENTING DIABETES

Type 1 diabetes cannot be prevented with current knowledge. Effective approaches are available to prevent type 2 diabetes and to prevent the complications and premature death that can result from all types of diabetes. These include policies and practices across whole populations and within specific settings (school, home, workplace) that contribute to good health for everyone, regardless of whether they have diabetes, such as exercising regularly, eating healthily, avoiding smoking, and controlling blood pressure and lipids.

Taking a life-course perspective is essential for preventing type 2 diabetes, as it is for many health conditions. Early in life, when eating and physical activity habits are formed and when the long-term regulation of energy balance may be programmed, there is a critical window for intervention to mitigate the risk of obesity and type 2 diabetes later in life.

No single policy or intervention can ensure this happens. It calls for a whole-of-government and whole-of-society approach, in which all sectors systematically consider the health impact of policies in trade, agriculture, finance, transport, education and urban planning – recognizing that health is enhanced or obstructed as a result of policies in these and other areas.

MANAGING DIABETES

The starting point for living well with diabetes is an early diagnosis – the longer a person lives with undiagnosed and untreated diabetes, the worse their health outcomes are likely to be. Easy access to basic diagnostics, such as blood glucose testing, should therefore be available in primary health-care settings. Established systems for referral and back-referral are needed, as patients will need periodic specialist assessment or treatment for complications.

For those who are diagnosed with diabetes, a series of cost-effective interventions can improve their outcomes, regardless of what type of diabetes they may have. These interventions include blood glucose control, through a combination of diet, physical activity and, if necessary, medication; control of blood pressure and lipids to reduce cardiovascular risk and other complications; and regular screening for damage to the eyes, kidneys and feet, to facilitate early treatment. Diabetes management can be strengthened through the use of standards and protocols.

Efforts to improve capacity for diagnosis and treatment of diabetes should occur in the context of integrated noncommunicable disease (NCD) management to yield better outcomes. At a minimum, diabetes and cardiovascular disease management can be combined. Integrated management of diabetes and tuberculosis and/or HIV/AIDS can be considered where there is high prevalence of these diseases.

NATIONAL CAPACITY FOR PREVENTION AND CONTROL OF DIABETES

National capacity to prevent and control diabetes as assessed in the 2015 NCD Country Capacity Survey varies widely by region and country-income level. Most countries report having national diabetes policies, as well as national policies to reduce key risk factors and national guidelines or protocols to improve management of diabetes. In some regions and among lower-income countries, however, these policies and guidelines lack funding and implementation.

In general, primary health-care practitioners in low-income countries do not have access to the basic technologies needed to help people with diabetes properly manage their disease. Only one in three low- and middle-income countries report that the most basic technologies for diabetes diagnosis and management are generally available in primary health-care facilities.

Many countries have conducted national population-based surveys of the prevalence of physical inactivity and overweight and obesity in the past 5 years, but less than half have included blood glucose measurement in these surveys.

ACCESS TO INSULIN AND OTHER ESSENTIAL MEDICINES

The lack of access to affordable insulin remains a key impediment to successful treatment and results in needless complications and premature deaths. Insulin and oral hypoglycaemic agents are reported as generally available in only a minority of low-income countries. Moreover, essential medicines critical to gaining control of diabetes, such as agents to lower blood pressure and lipid levels, are frequently unavailable in low- and middle-income countries. Policy and programme interventions are needed to improve equitable access.

CONCLUSIONS AND RECOMMENDATIONS

This first WHO *Global report on diabetes* underscores the enormous scale of the diabetes problem, and also the potential to reverse current trends. The political basis for concerted action to address diabetes is there, woven into the Sustainable Development Goals, the United Nations Political Declaration on NCDs, and the WHO NCD Global Action Plan. Where built upon, these foundations will catalyse action by all.

Countries can take a series of actions, in line with the objectives of the WHO NCD Global Action Plan 2013–2020, to reduce the impact of diabetes:

- Establish national mechanisms such as high-level multisectoral commissions to ensure political commitment, resource allocation, effective leadership and advocacy for an integrated NCD response, with specific attention to diabetes.

- Build the capacity of ministries of health to exercise a strategic leadership role, engaging stakeholders across sectors and society. Set national targets and indicators to foster accountability. Ensure that national policies and plans addressing diabetes are fully costed and then funded and implemented.

- Prioritize actions to prevent people becoming overweight and obese, beginning before birth and in early childhood. Implement policies and programmes to promote breastfeeding and the consumption of healthy foods and to discourage the consumption of unhealthy foods, such as sugary sodas. Create supportive built and social environments for physical activity. A combination of fiscal policies, legislation, changes to the environment and raising awareness of health risks works best for promoting healthier diets and physical activity at the necessary scale.

- Strengthen the health system response to NCDs, including diabetes, particularly at primary-care level. Implement guidelines and protocols to improve diagnosis and management of diabetes in primary health care. Establish policies and programmes to ensure equitable access to essential technologies for diagnosis and management. Make essential medicines such as human insulin available and affordable to all who need them.

- Address key gaps in the diabetes knowledge base. Outcome evaluations of innovative programmes intended to change behaviour are a particular need.

- Strengthen national capacity to collect, analyse and use representative data on the burden and trends of diabetes and its key risk factors. Develop, maintain and strengthen a diabetes registry if feasible and sustainable.

There are no simple solutions for addressing diabetes but coordinated, multicomponent intervention can make a significant difference. Everyone can play a role in reducing the impact of all forms of diabetes. Governments, health-care providers, people with diabetes, civil society, food producers and manufacturers and suppliers of medicines and technology are all stakeholders. Collectively, they can make a significant contribution to halt the rise in diabetes and improve the lives of those living with the disease.

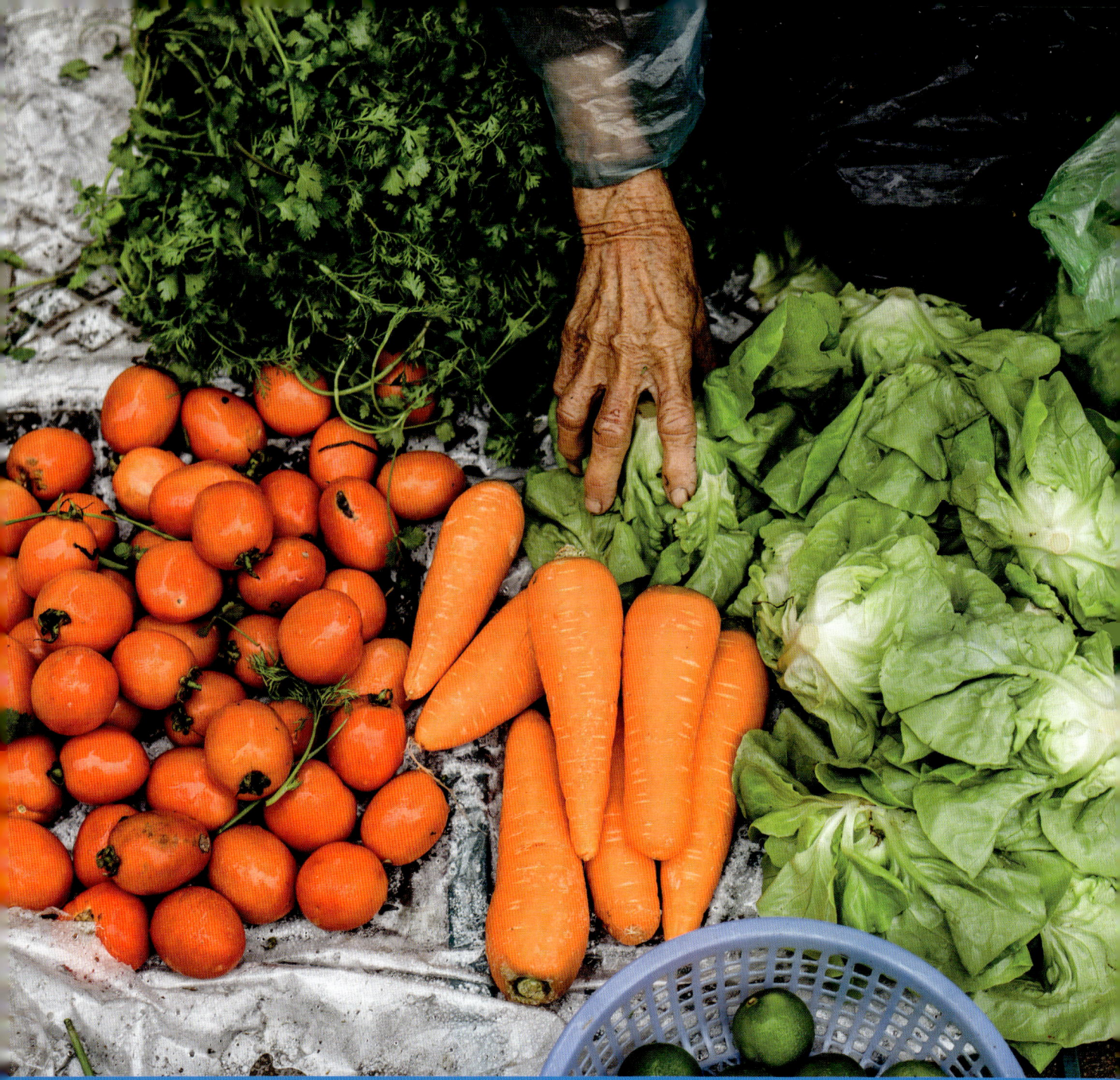

BACKGROUND

KEY MESSAGES

Diabetes is a chronic, progressive disease characterized by elevated levels of blood glucose.

Diabetes of all types can lead to complications in many parts of the body and can increase the overall risk of dying prematurely.

Countries have committed to halt the rise in diabetes, to reduce diabetes-related premature mortality and to improve access to essential diabetes medicines and basic technologies.

Effective tools are available to prevent type 2 diabetes and to improve management to reduce the complications and premature death that can result from all types of diabetes.

Diabetes is a serious, chronic disease that occurs either when the pancreas does not produce enough insulin (a hormone that regulates blood glucose), or when the body cannot effectively use the insulin it produces *(1)*. Raised blood glucose, a common effect of uncontrolled diabetes, may, over time, lead to serious damage to the heart, blood vessels, eyes, kidneys and nerves. More than 400 million people live with diabetes.

Type 1 diabetes (previously known as insulin-dependent, juvenile or childhood-onset diabetes) is characterized by deficient insulin production in the body. People with type 1 diabetes require daily administration of insulin to regulate the amount of glucose in their blood. If they do not have access to insulin, they cannot survive. The cause of type 1 diabetes is not known and it is currently not preventable. Symptoms include excessive urination and thirst, constant hunger, weight loss, vision changes and fatigue.

Type 2 diabetes (formerly called non-insulin-dependent or adult-onset diabetes) results from the body's ineffective use of insulin. Type 2 diabetes accounts for the vast majority of people with diabetes around the world *(1)*. Symptoms may be similar to those of type 1 diabetes, but are often less marked or absent. As a result, the disease may go undiagnosed for several years, until complications have already arisen. For many years type 2 diabetes was seen only in adults but it has begun to occur in children.

Impaired glucose tolerance (IGT) and **impaired fasting glycaemia (IFG)** are intermediate conditions in the transition between normal blood glucose levels and diabetes (especially type 2), though the transition is not inevitable. People with IGT or IFG are at increased risk of heart attacks and strokes.

Gestational diabetes (GDM) is a temporary condition that occurs in pregnancy and carries long-term risk of type 2 diabetes *(2)*. The condition is present when blood glucose values are above normal but still below those diagnostic of diabetes *(3)*. Women with gestational diabetes are at increased risk of some complications during pregnancy and delivery, as are their infants. Gestational diabetes is diagnosed through prenatal screening, rather than reported symptoms.

RISK FACTORS FOR DIABETES

Type 1. The exact causes of type 1 diabetes are unknown. It is generally agreed that type 1 diabetes is the result of a complex interaction between genes and environmental factors, though no specific environmental risk factors have been shown to cause a significant number of cases. The majority of type 1 diabetes occurs in children and adolescents.

Type 2. The risk of type 2 diabetes is determined by an interplay of genetic and metabolic factors. Ethnicity, family history of diabetes, and previous gestational diabetes combine with older age, overweight and obesity, unhealthy diet, physical inactivity and smoking to increase risk.

Excess body fat, a summary measure of several aspects of diet and physical activity, is the strongest risk factor for type 2 diabetes, both in terms of clearest evidence base and largest relative risk. Overweight and obesity, together with physical inactivity, are estimated to cause a large proportion of the global diabetes burden *(4)*. Higher waist circumference and higher body mass index (BMI) are associated with increased risk of type 2 diabetes, though the relationship may vary in different populations *(5)*. Populations in South-East Asia, for example, develop diabetes at a lower level of BMI than populations of European origin *(6)*.

Several dietary practices are linked to unhealthy body weight and/or type 2 diabetes risk, including high intake of saturated fatty acids, high total fat intake and inadequate consumption of dietary fibre *(7, 8, 9)*. High intake of sugar-sweetened beverages, which contain considerable amounts of free sugars,[1] increases the likelihood of being overweight or obese, particularly among children *(10, 11)*. Recent evidence further suggests an association between high consumption of sugar-sweetened beverages and increased risk of type 2 diabetes *(7, 12, 13, 14)*.

Early childhood nutrition affects the risk of type 2 diabetes later in life. Factors that appear to increase risk include poor fetal growth, low birth weight (particularly if followed by rapid postnatal catch-up growth) and high birth weight *(15, 16, 17, 18, 19, 20, 21)*.

Active (as distinct from passive) smoking increases the risk of type 2 diabetes, with the highest risk among heavy smokers *(22)*. Risk remains elevated for about

> **Overweight and obesity are the strongest risk factors for type 2 diabetes**

---

1. This includes "all monosaccharides and disaccharides added to foods by the manufacturer, cook, or consumer, plus sugars naturally present in honey, syrups, and fruit juices". Source: Joint WHO/FAO Expert Consultation, WHO Technical Report Series 916 Diet, Nutrition, and the Prevention of Chronic Diseases. Geneva, WHO, 2003.

10 years after smoking cessation, falling more quickly for lighter smokers *(23)*.

Gestational diabetes. Risk factors and risk markers for GDM include age (the older a woman of reproductive age is, the higher her risk of GDM); overweight or obesity; excessive weight gain during pregnancy; a family history of diabetes; GDM during a previous pregnancy; a history of stillbirth or giving birth to an infant with congenital abnormality; and excess glucose in urine during pregnancy *(24)*. Diabetes in pregnancy and GDM increase the risk of future obesity and type 2 diabetes in offspring.

COMPLICATIONS OF DIABETES

When diabetes is not well managed, complications develop that threaten health and endanger life. Acute complications are a significant contributor to mortality, costs and poor quality of life. Abnormally high blood glucose can have a life-threatening impact if it triggers conditions such as diabetic ketoacidosis (DKA) in types 1 and 2, and hyperosmolar coma in type 2. Abnormally low blood glucose can occur in all types of diabetes and may result in seizures or loss of consciousness. It may happen after skipping a meal or exercising more than usual, or if the dosage of anti-diabetic medication is too high.

Over time diabetes can damage the heart, blood vessels, eyes, kidneys and nerves, and increase the risk of heart disease and stroke. Such damage can result in reduced blood flow, which – combined with nerve damage (neuropathy) in the feet – increases the chance of foot ulcers, infection and the eventual need for limb amputation. Diabetic retinopathy is an important cause of blindness and occurs as a result of long-term accumulated damage to the small blood vessels in the retina. Diabetes is among the leading causes of kidney failure.

Uncontrolled diabetes in pregnancy can have a devastating effect on both mother and child, substantially increasing the risk of fetal loss, congenital malformations, stillbirth, perinatal death, obstetric complications, and maternal morbidity and mortality. Gestational diabetes increases the risk of some adverse outcomes for mother and offspring during pregnancy, childbirth and immediately after delivery (pre-eclampsia and eclampsia in the mother; large for gestational age and shoulder dystocia in the offspring) *(25)*. However, it is not known what proportion of obstructed births or maternal and perinatal deaths can be attributed to hyperglycaemia.

The combination of increasing prevalence of diabetes and increasing lifespans in many populations with diabetes may be leading to a changing spectrum of the types of morbidity that accompany diabetes. In addition to the traditional complications described above, diabetes has been associated with increased rates of specific cancers, and increased rates of physical and cognitive disability *(26)*. This diversification of complications and increased years of life spent with diabetes indicates a need to better monitor the quality of life of people with diabetes and assess

Diabetes can damage the heart, blood vessels, eyes, kidneys and nerves, leading to disability and premature death

the impact of interventions on quality of life.

ECONOMIC IMPACT OF DIABETES

Diabetes imposes a large economic burden on the global health-care system and the wider global economy. This burden can be measured through direct medical costs, indirect costs associated with productivity loss, premature mortality and the negative impact of diabetes on nations' gross domestic product (GDP).

Direct medical costs associated with diabetes include expenditures for preventing and treating diabetes and its complications. These include outpatient and emergency care; inpatient hospital care; medications and medical supplies such as injection devices and self-monitoring consumables; and long-term care.

Based on cost estimates from a recent systematic review, it has been estimated that the direct annual cost of diabetes to the world is more than US$ 827 billion *(27, 28)*. The International Diabetes Federation (IDF) estimates that total global health-care spending on diabetes more than tripled over the period 2003 to 2013 – the result of increases in the number of people with diabetes and increases in per capita diabetes spending *(29)*.

While the major diabetes cost drivers are hospital inpatient and outpatient care, a contributing factor to this increase is the rise in expenditure on patented, branded medicines used to treat people with diabetes, including both new oral treatments for type 2 diabetes and analogue insulins[1]. None of these preparations has yet been included in the WHO *Model list of essential medicines*,[2] because systematic evidence reviews find that they provide little or no advantage over cheaper generic alternatives *(30)*.

The increase in total global diabetes health expenditure is expected to continue. Low- and middle- income countries will carry a larger proportion of this future global health-care expenditure burden than high-income countries.

Catastrophic medical expenditure. Besides the economic burden on the health-care system and national economy, diabetes can impose a large economic burden on people with diabetes and their families in terms of higher out-of-pocket health-care payments and loss of family income associated with disability and premature loss of life.

The relationship between diabetes and the risk of catastrophic medical expenditure by individuals and families has been explored in 35 developing countries. This research found that people with diabetes had a significantly greater chance of incurring catastrophic medical expenditure compared to similar individuals without diabetes. Health insurance was not significantly related to lower risks of

> **People with diabetes are more likely to incur catastrophic personal health expenditure**

---

1. These are insulins derived from human insulin by modifying its structure to change the pharmacokinetic profile.

2. WHO's *Model list of essential medicines* comprises a set of medicines that satisfy the priority health-care needs of the population, meaning they should be available at all times, in adequate amounts and in appropriate dosage forms, at a price the community can afford.

catastrophic medical expenditure. The effects were more marked in lower-income countries *(31)*.

Impact on national economies. One study estimates that losses in GDP worldwide from 2011 to 2030, including both the direct and indirect costs of diabetes, will total US$ 1.7 trillion, comprising US$ 900 billion for high-income countries and US$ 800 billion for low- and middle-income countries *(32)*.

DIABETES AND THE GLOBAL PUBLIC HEALTH AGENDA

Diabetes is recognized as an important cause of premature death and disability. It is one of four priority noncommunicable diseases (NCDs) targeted by world leaders in the 2011 Political Declaration on the Prevention and Control of NCDs *(33)*. The declaration recognizes that the incidence and impacts of diabetes and other NCDs can be largely prevented or reduced with an approach that incorporates evidence-based, affordable, cost-effective, population-wide and multisectoral interventions. To catalyse national action, the World Health Assembly adopted a comprehensive global monitoring framework in 2013, comprised of nine voluntary global targets to reach by 2025 (see Box 1, page 16). This was accompanied by the WHO *Global action plan for the prevention and control of NCDs 2013–2020* (WHO NCD Global Action Plan), endorsed by the 66th World Health Assembly *(34)*, which provides a roadmap and policy options to attain the nine voluntary global targets. Diabetes and its key risk factors are strongly reflected in the targets and indicators of the global monitoring framework and the WHO NCD Global Action Plan.

These commitments were deepened in 2015 by the United Nations General Assembly's adoption of the 2030 Agenda for Sustainable Development *(35)*. In this context, countries have agreed to take action to achieve ambitious targets by 2030 – to reduce premature mortality from NCDs by one-third; to achieve universal health coverage; and to provide access to affordable essential medicines.

To halt the rise in obesity and type 2 diabetes it is imperative to scale-up population-level prevention. Policy measures are needed to increase access to affordable, healthy foods and beverages; to promote physical activity; and to reduce exposure to tobacco. Mass media campaigns and social marketing can influence positive change and make healthy behaviours more the norm. These strategies have the potential to reduce the occurrence of type 2 diabetes and may also reduce complications associated with diabetes.

To reduce avoidable mortality from diabetes and improve outcomes, access to affordable treatment is critical. Lack of access to insulin in many countries and communities remains a critical impediment to successful treatment efforts. Inadequate access to oral hypoglycaemic medication, and medication to control blood pressure and lipids, is also a barrier. Improved management in primary care with ongoing support by community health workers can lead to better control of diabetes and fewer complications.

This report builds on ongoing global work to address NCDs. It aims to draw focused attention to the

Diabetes is 1 of 4 priority NCDs targeted by world leaders

public health challenge of diabetes and to generate momentum for national, regional and global action. Part 1 presents an overview of the global prevalence of diabetes, the burden of mortality related to blood glucose, and what is known about the extent of diabetes-related complications. Part 2 reviews evidence for action to prevent type 2 diabetes through population-wide and targeted interventions. Part 3 discusses diagnosis and early detection of diabetes, along with actions required to improve outcomes for those living with it. Part 4 gives the current status of national responses to diabetes and provides data on efforts to monitor, prevent and manage it (diabetes country profiles are available at *www.who.int/diabetes/global-report*). The final section presents conclusions and recommendations for realizing the global commitments made to prevent diabetes and reduce its health impact.

BOX 1. VOLUNTARY GLOBAL TARGETS FOR PREVENTION AND CONTROL OF NONCOMMUNICABLE DISEASES TO BE ATTAINED BY 2025

(1) A 25% relative reduction in the overall mortality from cardiovascular diseases, cancer, diabetes, or chronic respiratory diseases

(2) At least 10% relative reduction in the harmful use of alcohol, as appropriate, within the national context

(3) A 10% relative reduction in prevalence of insufficient physical activity

(4) A 30% relative reduction in mean population intake of salt/sodium

(5) A 30% relative reduction in prevalence of current tobacco use

(6) A 25% relative reduction in the prevalence of raised blood pressure or contain the prevalence of raised blood pressure, according to national circumstances

(7) Halt the rise in diabetes and obesity

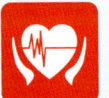
(8) At least 50% of eligible people receive drug therapy and counselling (including glycaemic control) to prevent heart attacks and strokes

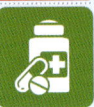
(9) An 80% availability of the affordable basic technologies and essential medicines, including generics, required to treat major noncommunicable diseases in both public and private facilities

Source: (34).

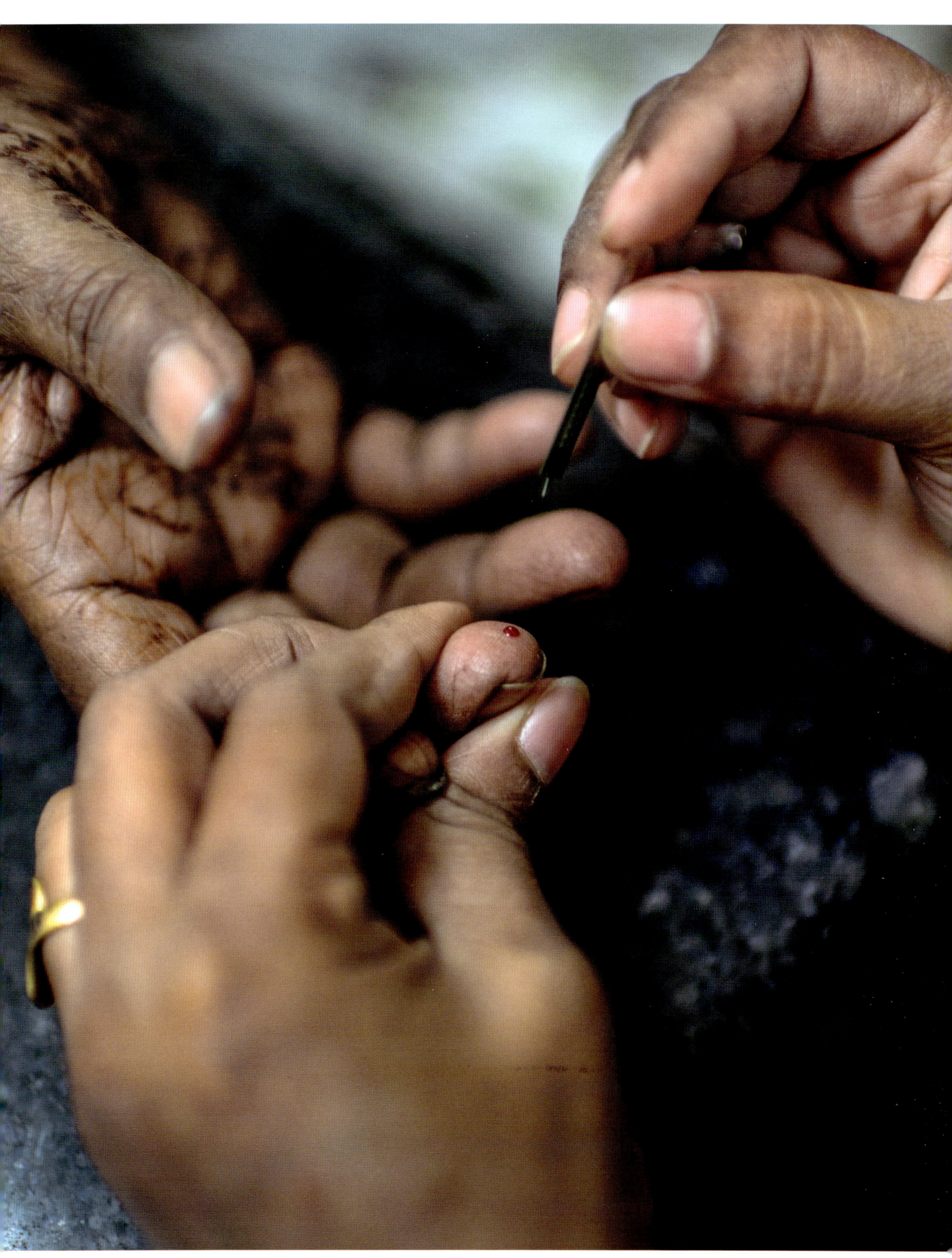

REFERENCES

1. Definition, Diagnosis and Classification of Diabetes Mellitus and its Complications. Part 1: Diagnosis and Classification of Diabetes Mellitus (WHO/NCD/NCS/99.2). Geneva: World Health Organization; 1999.

2. Bellamy L, Casas JP, Hingorani AD, Williams D. Type 2 diabetes mellitus after gestational diabetes: a systematic review and meta-analysis. Lancet. 2009;373:1773–1779.

3. Diagnostic criteria and classification of hyperglycaemia first detected in pregnancy (WHO/NMH/MND/13.2). Geneva: World Health Organization; 2013.

4. GBD 2013 Risk Factors Collaborators. Global, regional, and national comparative risk assessment of 79 behavioural, environmental and occupational, and metabolic risks or clusters of risks in 188 countries, 1990–2013: a systematic analysis for the Global Burden of Disease Study 2013. Lancet. 2015;386(10010):2287–323.

5. Vazquez G, Duval S, Jacobs DR Jr, Silventoinen K. Comparison of body mass index, waist circumference and waist/hip ratio in predicting incident diabetes: a meta-analysis. Epidemiologic Reviews. 2007;29:115–28.

6. Ramachandran A, Ma RC, Snehalatha C. Diabetes in Asia. Lancet. 2010;375:(9712)408–418.

7. Ley SH, Hamdy, O, Mohan V, Hu FB. Prevention and management of type 2 diabetes: dietary components and nutritional strategies. Lancet. 2014;383(9933):1999–2007.

8. Fats and fatty acids in human nutrition: report of an expert consultation. FAO Food and Nutrition Paper 91. Rome: Food and Agriculture Organization of the United Nations; 2010.

9. Diet, nutrition and the prevention of chronic diseases: report of a Joint WHO/FAO Expert Consultation. WHO Technical Report Series, No. 916. Geneva: World Health Organization; 2003.

10. WHO Guideline: sugars intake in adults and children. Geneva: World Health Organization; 2015.

11. Te Morenga L, Mallard S, Mann J. Dietary sugars and body weight: systematic review and meta analyses of randomised controlled trials and cohort studies. British Medical Journal. 2013;346:e7492.

12. Imamura F, O'Connor L, Ye Z, Mursu J, Hayashino Y, Bhupathiraju SN, Forouhi NG. Consumption of sugar-sweetened beverages, artificially sweetened beverages, and fruit juice and incidence of type 2 diabetes: systematic review, meta-analysis, and estimation of population attributable fraction. British Medical Journal. 2015;351:h3576.

13. The InterAct consortium. Consumption of sweet beverages and type 2 diabetes incidence in European adults: results from EPIC-InterAct. Diabetologia. 2013;56:1520–30.

14. Malik VS, Popkin BM, Bray GA, Després J-P, Willett WC, Hu FB. Sugar-sweetened beverages and risk of metabolic syndrome and type 2 diabetes: a meta-analysis. Diabetes Care. 2010;33:2477–83.

15. Policy brief: Global nutrition targets 2025: Childhood overweight. Geneva: World Health Organization; 2014.

16. Nolan C, Damm P, Prentki Ml. Type 2 diabetes across generations: from pathophysiology to prevention and management. Lancet. 2011;378(9786):169–181.

17. Darnton-Hill I, Nishida C, James WPT. A life-course approach to diet, nutrition and the prevention of chronic diseases. Public Health Nutrition. 2004;7(1A):101–21.

18. Diet, nutrition and the prevention of chronic diseases. Report of a Joint WHO/FAO Expert Consultation. Geneva: World Health Organization; 2003.

19. Johnsson, IW, Haglund B, Ahlsson F, Gustafsson J. A high birth weight is associated with increased risk of type 2 diabetes and obesity. Pediatric Obesity. 2015;10(2):77–83.

20. Whincup PH, Kaye SJ, Owen CG, et al. Birth weight and risk of type 2 diabetes: a systematic review. Journal of the American Medical Association. 2008;300:2886–2897.

21. Harder T, Rodekamp E, Schellong K, Dudenhausen JW, Plagemann A. Birth weight and subsequent risk of type 2 diabetes: a meta-analysis. American Journal of Epidemiology. 2007;165:849–857.

22. Willi C, Bodenmann P, Ghali WA, Faris PD, Cornuz J. Active smoking and the risk of type 2 diabetes: a systematic review and meta-analysis. Journal of the American Medical Association. 2007;298:(22)2654–2664.

23. Luo J, Rossouw J, Tong E, Giovino GA, Lee CC, Chen C, et al. Smoking and diabetes: does the increased risk ever go away? American Journal of Epidemiology. 2013;178:(6)937–945.

24. Anna V, van der Ploeg HP, Cheung NW, Huxley RR, Bauman AE. Socio-demographic correlates of the increasing trend in prevalence of gestational diabetes mellitus in a large population of women between 1995 and 2005. Diabetes Care. 2008;31:(12)2288–2293.

25. Wendland EM, Torloni MR, Falavigna M, Trujillo J, Dode MA, Campos MA, et al. Gestational diabetes and pregnancy outcomes – a systematic review of the World Health Organization (WHO) and the International Association of Diabetes in Pregnancy Study Groups (IADPSG) diagnostic criteria. BMC Pregnancy Childbirth. 2012;12:(1)23.

26. Wong E, Backholer K, Gearon E, Harding J, Freak-Poli R, Stevenson C, et al. Diabetes and risk of physical disability in adults: a systematic review and meta-analysis. Lancet Diabetes Endocrinology. 2013;1:(2)106–114.

27. NCD Risk Factor Collaboration (NCD-RisC). Worldwide trends in diabetes since 1980: a pooled analysis of 751 population-based studies with 4*4 million participants. Lancet 2016; published online April 7. http://dx.doi.org/10.1016/S0140-6736(16)00618-8.

28. Seuring T, Archangelidi O, Suhrcke M. The economic costs of type 2 diabetes: A global systematic review. PharmacoEconomics. 2015; 33(8): 811–31.

29. IDF Diabetes Atlas, 6th ed. Brussels, International Diabetes Federation; 2013.

30. Singh SR, Ahmad F, Lal A, Yu C, Bai Z, Bennett H. Efficacy and safety of insulin analogues for the management of diabetes mellitus: a meta-analysis. Canadian Medical Association Journal. 2009;180: (4)385–397.

31. Smith-Spangler CM, Bhattacharya J, Goldhaber-Fiebert JD. Diabetes, its treatment, and catastrophic medical spending in 35 developing countries. Diabetes Care. 2012;35:(2)319–326.

32. Bloom DE, Cafiero ET, Jané-Llopis E, Abrahams-Gessel S, Bloom LR, Fathima S, et al. The global economic burden of noncommunicable diseases (Working Paper Series). Geneva: Harvard School of Public Health and World Economic Forum; 2011.

33. Resolution 66/2. Political Declaration of the High-Level Meeting of the General Assembly on the Prevention and Control of Noncommunicable Diseases. In Sixty-sixth session ofthe United Nations General Assembly. New York: United Nations; 2011.

34. Global action plan for the prevention and control of noncommunicable diseases 2013-2020. Geneva: World Health Organization; 2013.

35. Transforming our world: the 2030 Agenda for Sustainable Development (A/RES/70/1). New York: United Nations General Assembly; 2015.

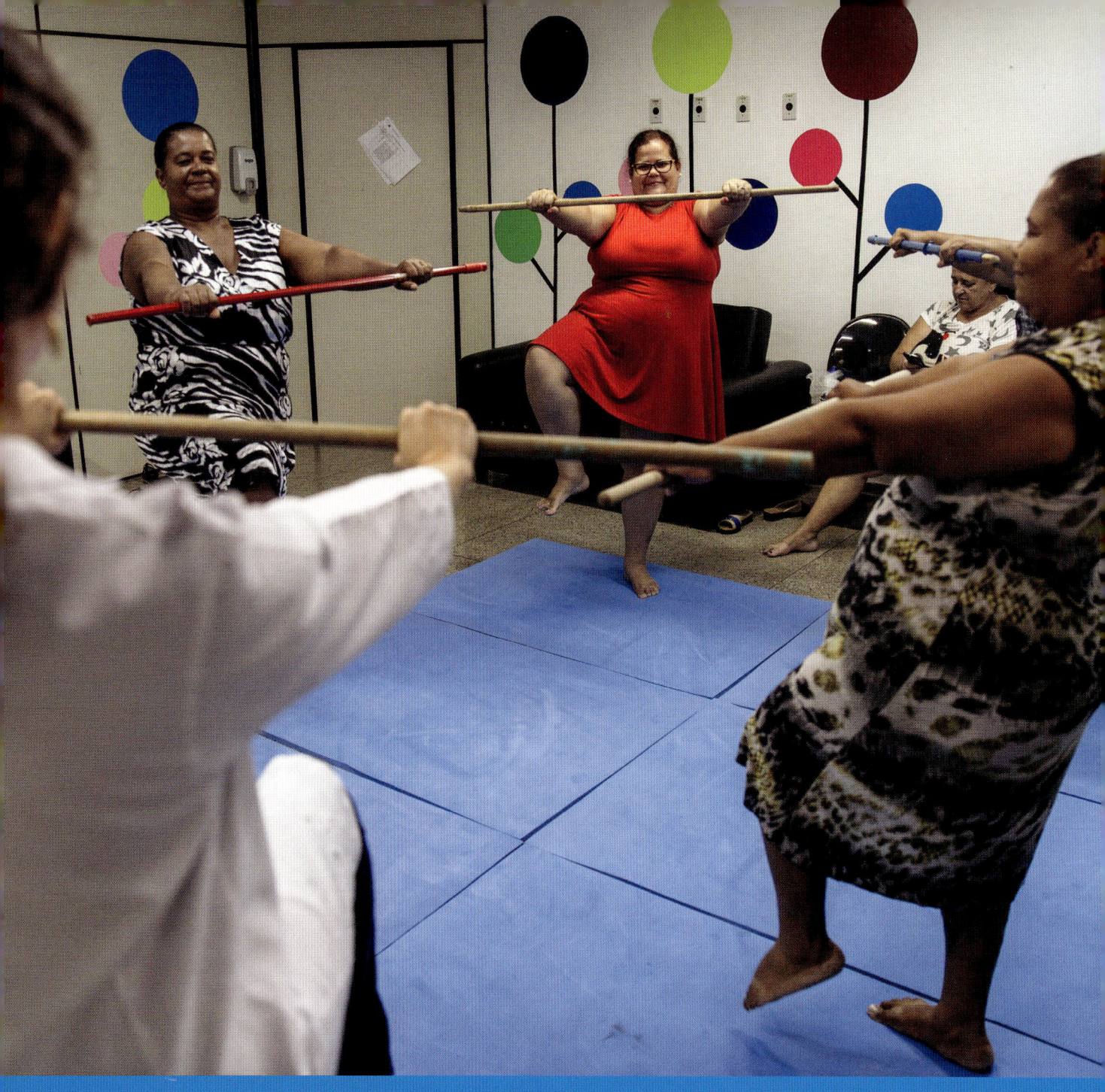

PART 1

GLOBAL BURDEN OF DIABETES

KEY MESSAGES

Diabetes caused 1.5 million deaths in 2012.

Higher-than-optimal blood glucose was responsible for an additional 2.2 million deaths as a result of increased risks of cardiovascular and other diseases, for a total of 3.7 million deaths related to blood glucose levels in 2012.

Many of these deaths (43%) occur under the age of 70.

In 2014, 422 million people in the world had diabetes – a prevalence of 8.5% among the adult population.

The prevalence of diabetes has been steadily increasing for the past 3 decades and is growing most rapidly in low- and middle-income countries.

Associated risk factors such as being overweight or obese are increasing.

Diabetes is an important cause of blindness, kidney failure, lower limb amputation and other long-term consequences that impact significantly on quality of life.

1.1 MORTALITY FROM HIGH BLOOD GLUCOSE, INCLUDING DIABETES

In 2012 there were 1.5 million deaths worldwide directly caused by diabetes. It was the eighth leading cause of death among both sexes and the fifth leading cause of death in women in 2012 (1).

Blood glucose levels that are higher-than-optimal, even if below the diagnostic threshold for diabetes, are a major source of mortality and morbidity. The diagnostic criterion for diabetes is fasting plasma glucose ≥ 7.0 mmol/L – a diagnostic point selected on the basis of micro-vascular complications such as diabetic retinopathy. The risk of macro-vascular disease, such as heart attack or stroke, however, starts increasing well before this diagnostic point (2, 3). To better understand the full impact of blood glucose levels on mortality therefore requires a look at mortality related to blood glucose as a risk factor.

The total burden of deaths from high blood glucose[1] in 2012 has been estimated to amount to 3.7 million. This number includes 1.5 million diabetes deaths, and an additional 2.2 million deaths from

---

1. **High blood glucose** is defined as a distribution of fasting plasma glucose in a population that is higher than the theoretical distribution that would minimize risks to health (derived from epidemiological studies). Further details on the values used to calculate the estimates presented here can be found in (2). High blood glucose is a statistical concept, not a clinical or diagnostic category.

FIGURE 1. PERCENTAGE OF ALL-CAUSE DEATHS ATTRIBUTED TO HIGH BLOOD GLUCOSE, BY AGE AND COUNTRY INCOME GROUP,[a] 2012 (A) MEN, (B) WOMEN

A (MEN)

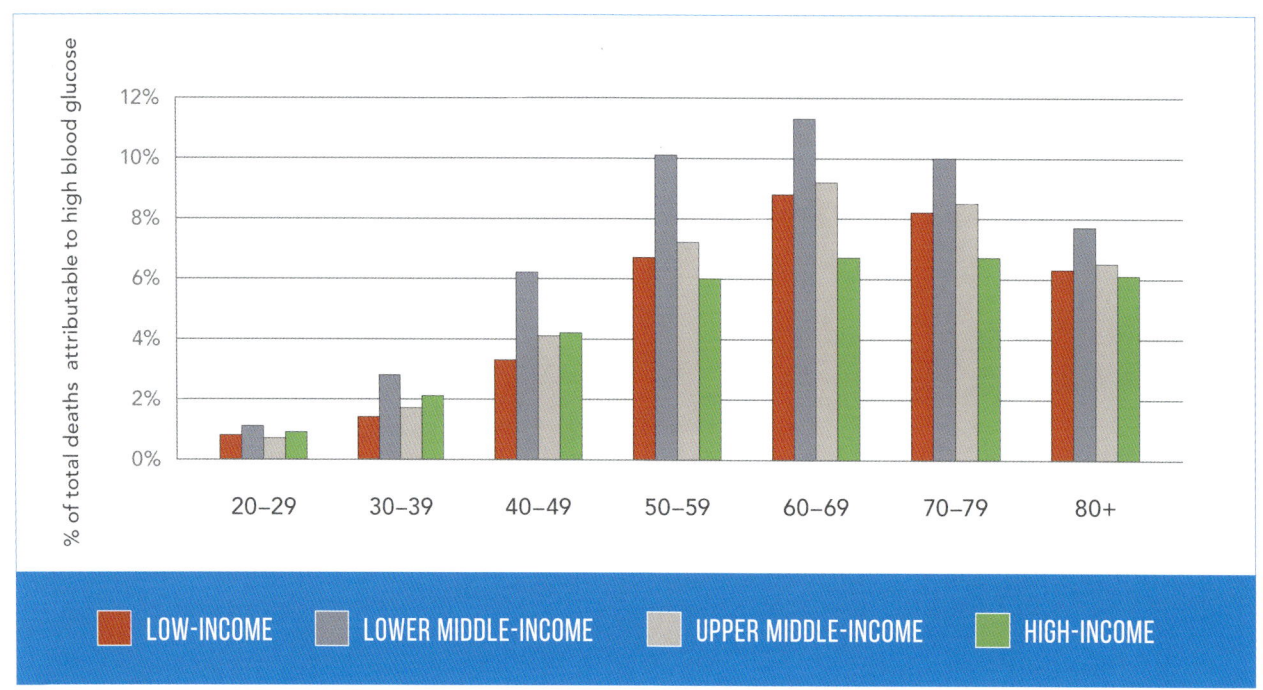

B (WOMEN)

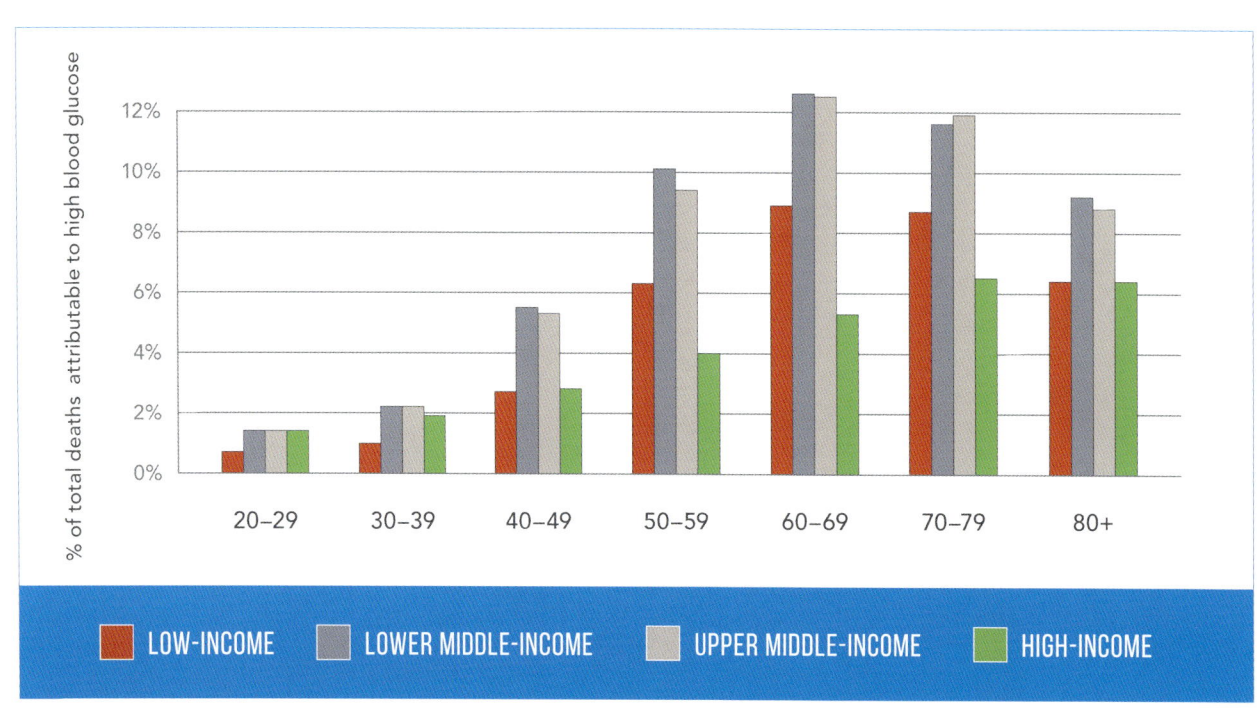

a. As categorized by the World Bank for 2012.

cardiovascular diseases, chronic kidney disease, and tuberculosis related to higher-than-optimal blood glucose. Its magnitude highlights that high blood glucose causes a large burden of mortality beyond those deaths directly caused by diabetes. The largest number of deaths resulting from high blood glucose occur in upper-middle income countries (1.5 million) and the lowest number in low-income countries (0.3 million).

After the age of 50, middle-income countries have the highest proportion of deaths attributed to high blood glucose, for both men and women (see Figure 1). Except in high-income countries, the proportion of deaths attributable to high blood glucose for both men and women are highest in the age group 60–69 years.

Forty-three per cent of all deaths attributable to high blood glucose occur prematurely, before the age of 70 years – an estimated 1.6 million deaths worldwide. Globally, high blood glucose causes about 7% of deaths among men aged 20–69 and 8% among women aged 20–69. Figure 2 shows that the percentage of premature deaths attributable to high blood glucose is higher in low- and middle-income countries than in high-income countries, and higher among men than women.

High blood glucose age-standardized mortality rates,

43% of all deaths due to high blood glucose occur before the age of 70

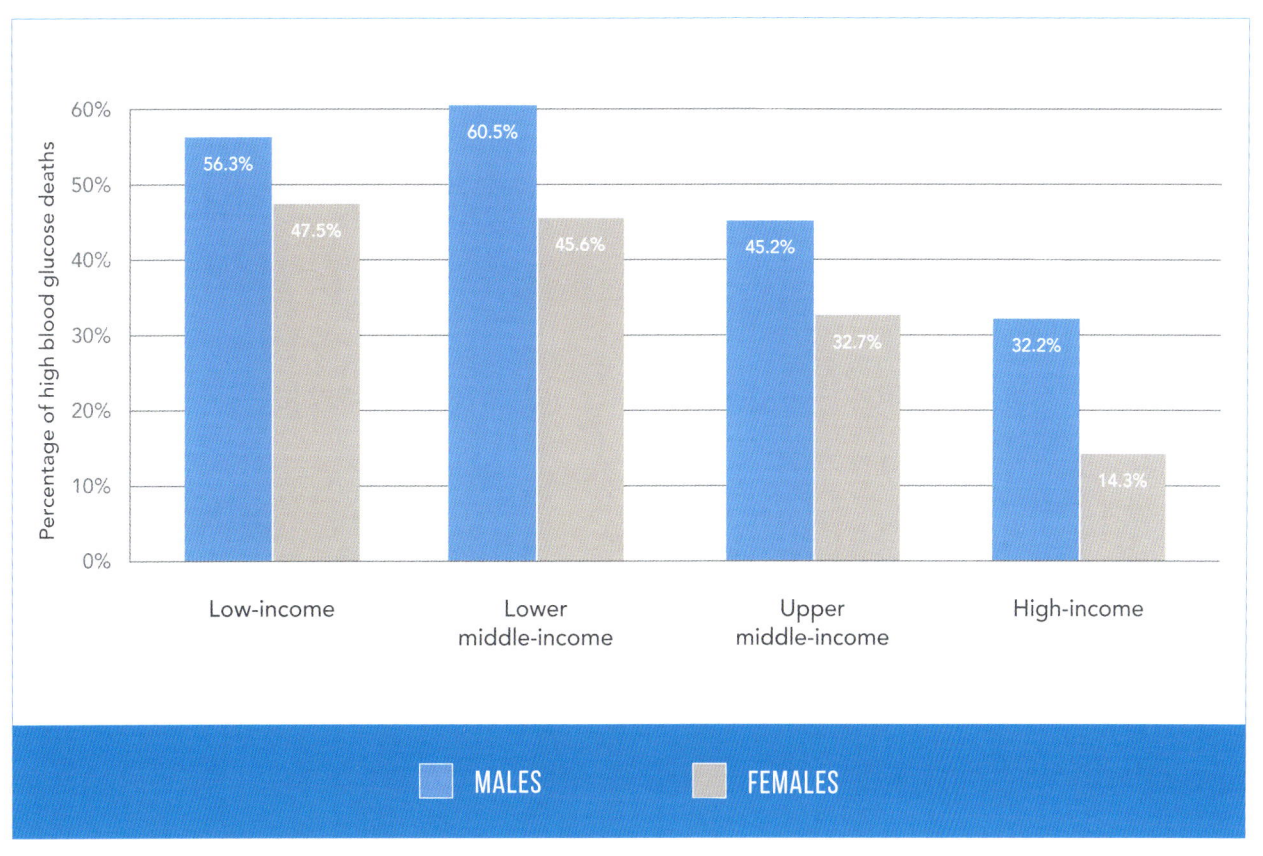

FIGURE 2. PERCENTAGE OF DEATHS ATTRIBUTED TO HIGH BLOOD GLUCOSE THAT OCCUR AT AGES 20–69 YEARS, BY SEX AND COUNTRY INCOME GROUP, 2012

which account for differences in population structure, are highly variable across WHO regions (Table 1). Rates are highest in the WHO Eastern Mediterranean, South-East Asia, and African Regions, and much lower in the remaining regions. In the WHO European and South-East Asia Regions and the Region of the Americas, high blood glucose mortality rates are considerably higher for men than for women.

During the period 2000–2012 the proportion of premature deaths

TABLE 1. HIGH BLOOD GLUCOSE AGE-STANDARDIZED MORTALITY RATES PER 100 000 BY WHO REGION, AGE 20+

	Both sexes	Female	Male
African Region	111.3	110.9	111.1
Region of the Americas	72.6	63.9	82.8
Eastern Mediterranean Region	139.6	140.2	138.3
European Region	55.7	46.5	64.5
South-East Asia Region	115.3	101.8	129.1
Western Pacific Region	67	65.8	67.8

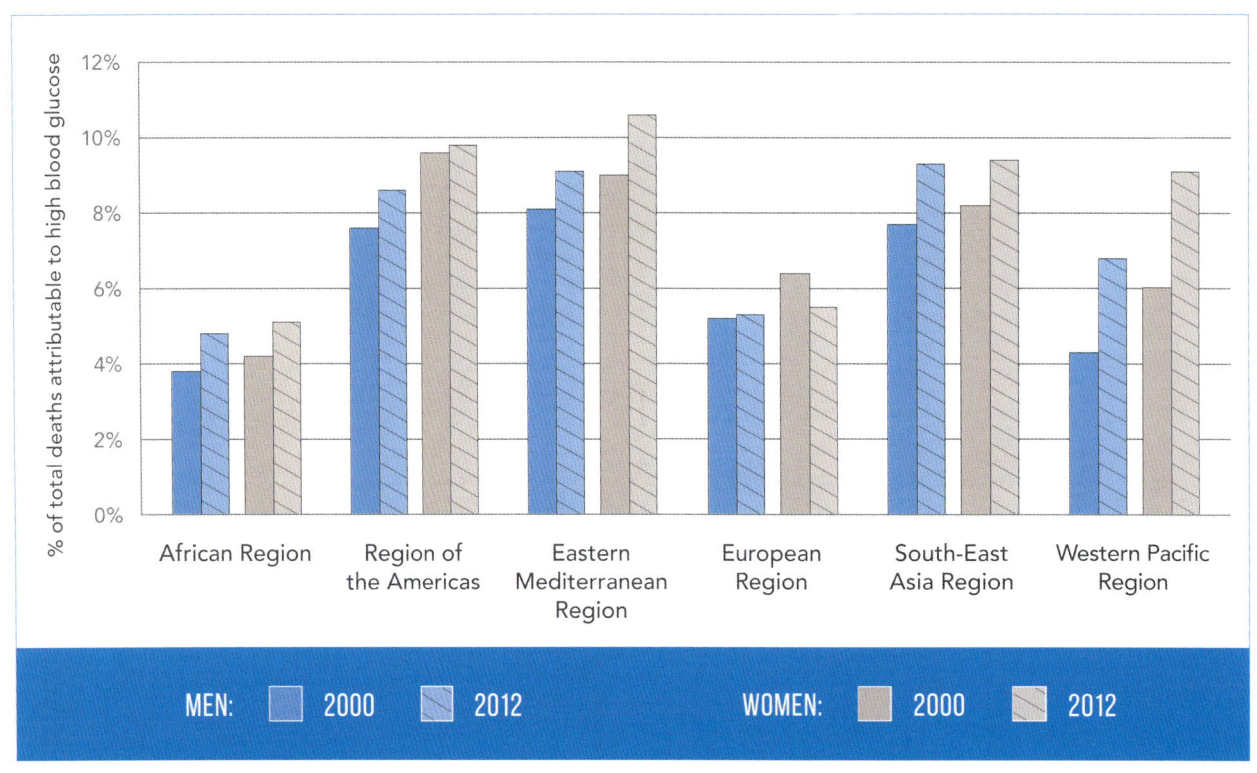

FIGURE 3. PERCENTAGE OF ALL DEATHS ATTRIBUTABLE TO HIGH BLOOD GLUCOSE FOR ADULTS AGED 20–69 YEARS, BY WHO REGION AND SEX, FOR YEARS 2000 AND 2012

(ages 20–69) attributable to high blood glucose increased for both sexes across all WHO regions, except among women in the WHO European Region (Figure 3). The increase in the proportion of deaths attributable to high blood glucose was highest in the WHO Western Pacific Region, where the total number of deaths attributable to high blood glucose during this period also increased from 490 000 to 944 000.

1.2 PREVALENCE OF DIABETES AND ASSOCIATED RISK FACTORS

WHO estimates that, globally, 422 million adults aged over 18 years were living with diabetes in 2014 (more details on methodology can be found in Annex B and reference 4). The largest numbers of people with diabetes were estimated for the WHO South-East Asia and Western Pacific Regions (see Table 2), accounting for approximately half the diabetes cases in the world.

The number of people with diabetes (defined in surveys as those having a fasting plasma glucose value of greater than or equal to 7.0 mmol/L or on medication for diabetes/raised blood glucose) has steadily risen over the past few decades, due to population growth, the increase in the average age of the population, and the rise in prevalence of diabetes at each age. Worldwide, the number of people with diabetes has substantially increased between 1980 and 2014, rising from 108 million to current numbers that are around four times higher (see Table 2). Forty per cent of this increase is estimated to result from population growth and ageing, 28% from a rise in age-specific prevalences, and 32% from the interaction of the two *(4)*.

In 2014

422 million

adults had diabetes

TABLE 2. ESTIMATED PREVALENCE AND NUMBER OF PEOPLE WITH DIABETES (ADULTS 18+ YEARS)

WHO Region	Prevalence (%)		Number (millions)	
	1980	2014	1980	2014
African Region	3.1%	7.1%	4	25
Region of the Americas	5%	8.3%	18	62
Eastern Mediterranean Region	5.9%	13.7%	6	43
European Region	5.3%	7.3%	33	64
South-East Asia Region	4.1%	8.6%	17	96
Western Pacific Region	4.4%	8.4%	29	131
Total[a]	**4.7%**	**8.5%**	**108**	**422**

a. Totals include non-Member States.

Source: (4).

Diabetes prevalence has doubled since 1980

In the past 3 decades the prevalence[1] (age-standardized) of diabetes has risen substantially in countries at all income levels, mirroring the global increase in the number of people who are overweight or obese. The global prevalence of diabetes has grown from 4.7% in 1980 to 8.5% in 2014, during which time prevalence has increased or at best remained unchanged in every country *(4)*. Over the past decade, diabetes prevalence has risen faster in low- and middle-income countries than in high-income countries (see Figure 4a). The WHO Eastern Mediterranean Region has experienced the greatest rise in diabetes prevalence, and is now the WHO region with the highest prevalence (13.7%) (see Figure 4b).

---

1. Unless otherwise noted, prevalence estimates reported in this section are age-standardized.

TYPE 1 DIABETES

Distinguishing between type 1 and type 2 diabetes is not always easy as it often requires relatively sophisticated laboratory tests for pancreas function. Distinct global estimates of diabetes prevalence for type 1 and type 2 therefore do not exist.

Much of our knowledge of the incidence of type 1 diabetes relates to children and has been generated by collaborative initiatives to develop population-based, standardized registries of new cases worldwide, such as the WHO DIAMOND Project *(5)*. Globally, these registries recorded large differences in the incidence and prevalence of type 1 diabetes, ranging from over 60 to under 0.5 cases annually per 100 000 children aged under 15 years; differences in case ascertainment

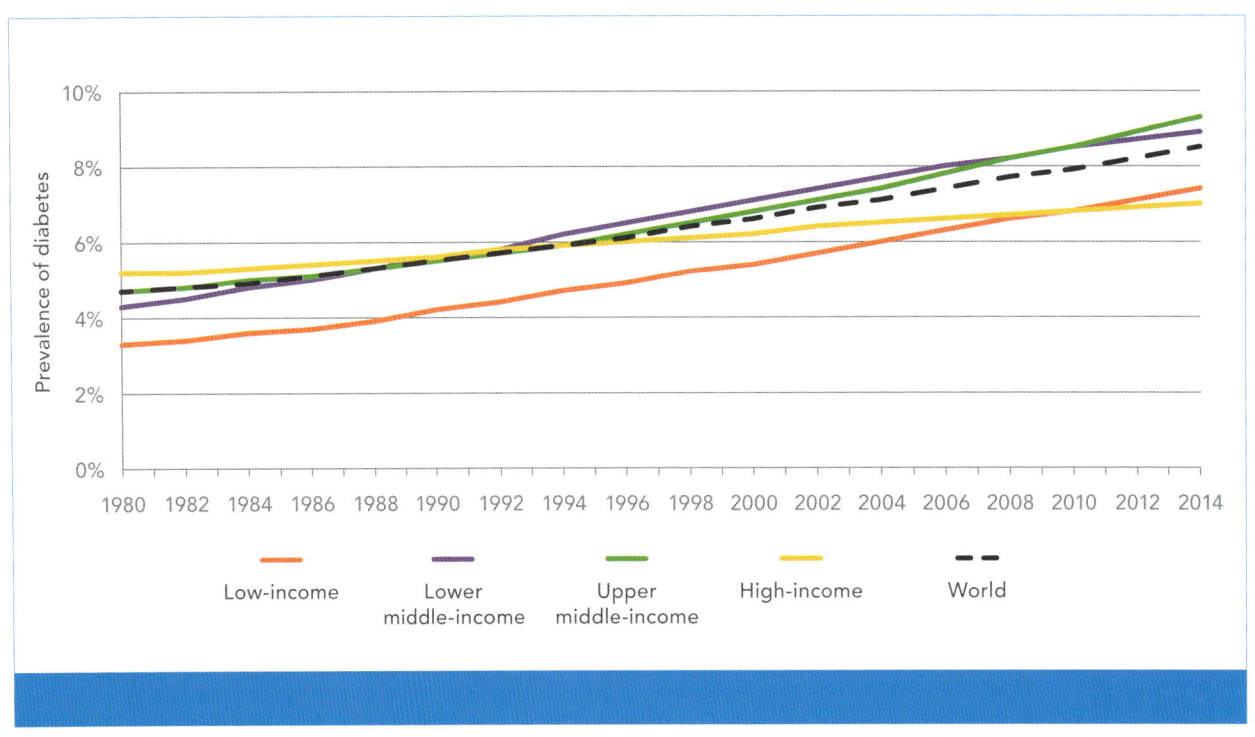

FIGURE 4A. TRENDS IN PREVALENCE OF DIABETES, 1980–2014, BY COUNTRY INCOME GROUP

may have contributed to the variability. Of the study sites in the WHO DIAMOND project, type 1 diabetes is most common in Scandinavian populations and in Sardinia and Kuwait, and much less common in Asia and Latin America *(6)*. Data are generally lacking for sub-Saharan Africa and large parts of Latin America. In the past few decades the annual incidence appears to be rising steadily by about 3% in high-income countries *(7, 8, 9)*.

TYPE 2 DIABETES AND GESTATIONAL DIABETES

Previously seen mainly in middle-aged and elderly people, type 2 diabetes occurs increasingly frequently in children and young people. Type 2 diabetes is often undiagnosed and studies to assess the number of newly occurring cases are complicated and consequently there are almost no data on true incidence. In high-income countries the prevalence of type 2 diabetes is frequently highest among people who are poor *(10)*. There are few data on the income gradient of diabetes in low- and middle-income countries, but data that exist suggest that although the prevalence of diabetes is often highest among wealthy people, this trend is reversing in some middle-income countries *(10)*.

The proportion of undiagnosed type 2 diabetes varies widely – a recent review of data from seven countries found that between 24%

FIGURE 4B. TRENDS IN PREVALENCE OF DIABETES, 1980–2014, BY WHO REGION

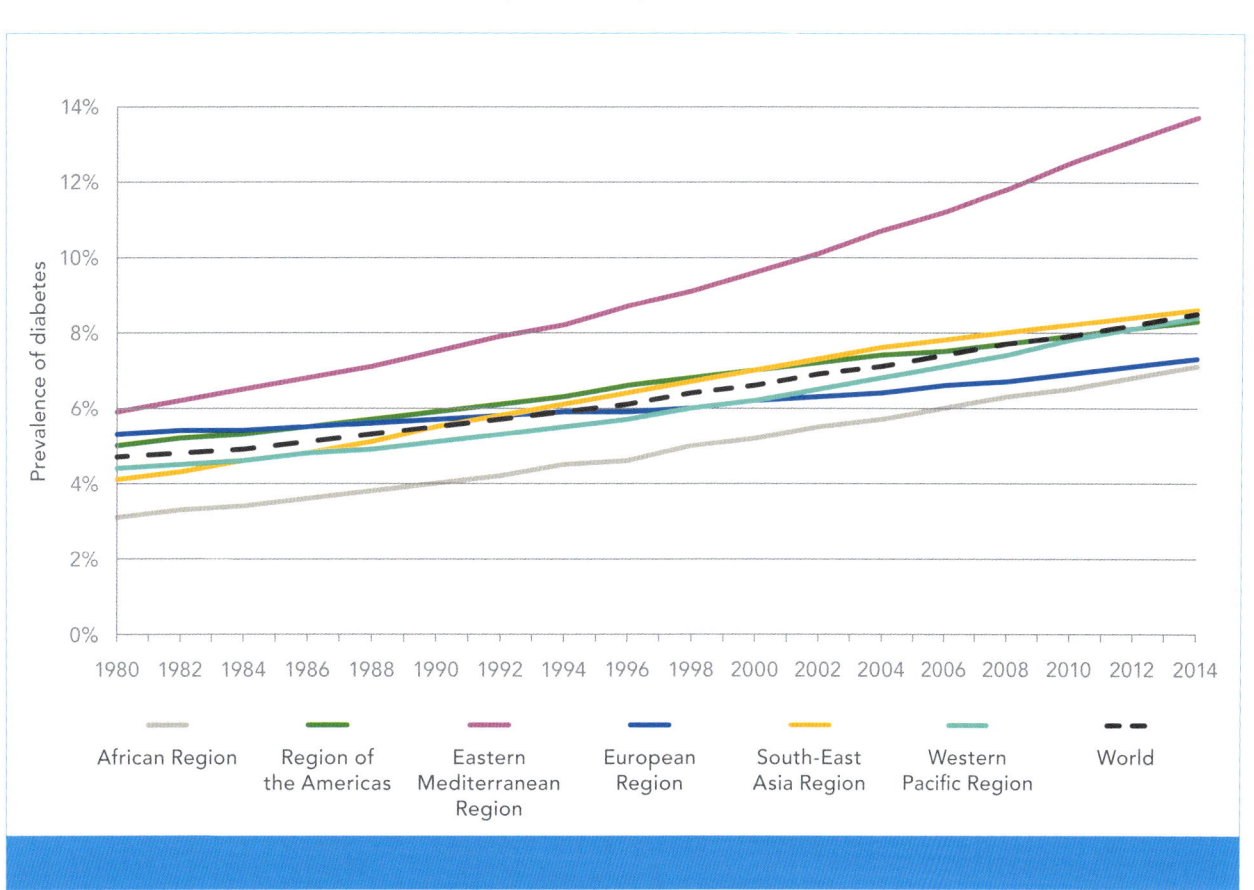

and 62% of people with diabetes were undiagnosed and untreated *(11)*. Analysis of data from WHO-supported STEPS surveys in 11 countries underscores the wide variation in the proportion of people undiagnosed and untreated: among people whose measured blood glucose was at or above the diagnostic threshold for diabetes, between 6% and 70% had been diagnosed with diabetes, and between 4% and 66% were taking medication to lower their blood glucose *(12)*. Even in high-income countries the proportion of undiagnosed diabetes can be as high as 30–50% *(13)*.

The frequency of previously undiagnosed diabetes in pregnancy and gestational diabetes varies among populations but probably affects 10–25% of pregnancies *(14)*. It has been estimated that most (75–90%) of cases of high blood glucose during pregnancy are gestational diabetes *(15)*.

ASSOCIATED RISK FACTORS

Regular physical activity reduces the risk of diabetes and raised blood glucose, and is an important contributor to overall energy balance, weight control and obesity prevention – all risk exposures linked to future diabetes prevalence *(16)*. The global target of a 10% relative reduction in physical inactivity is therefore strongly associated with the global target of halting the risk in diabetes.

However, the prevalence of physical inactivity globally is of increasing concern. In 2010, the latest year for which data are available, just under a quarter of all adults aged over 18 years did not meet the minimum recommendation for physical activity per week and were classified as insufficiently physically active *(16)*. In all WHO regions and across all country income groups women were less active than men, with 27% of women and 20% of men classified as insufficiently physically active. Physical inactivity is alarmingly common among adolescents, with 84% of girls and 78% of boys not meeting minimum requirements for physical activity for this age. The prevalence of physical inactivity is highest in high-income countries where it is almost double that of low-income countries. Among WHO regions, the Eastern Mediterranean Region showed the highest prevalence of inactivity in both adults and adolescents.

Being overweight or obese is strongly linked to diabetes. Despite the global voluntary target to halt the rise in obesity by 2025 *(16, 17)*, being overweight or obese has increased in almost all countries. In 2014, the latest year for which global estimates are available, more than one in three adults aged over 18 years were overweight and more than one in 10 were obese. Women were more overweight or obese than men. The prevalence of obesity was highest in the WHO Region of the Americas and lowest in the WHO South-East Asian Region (see Figure 5a). The proportion of people who are overweight or obese increases with country income level. High- and middle-income countries have more than double the overweight and obesity prevalence of low-income countries (see Figure 5b).

> **More than 1 in 3 adults were overweight and more than 1 in 10 were obese in 2014**

FIGURE 5A. PREVALENCE OF BEING OVERWEIGHT (BMI 25+) IN ADULTS OVER 18 YEARS, 2014, BY SEX AND WHO REGION

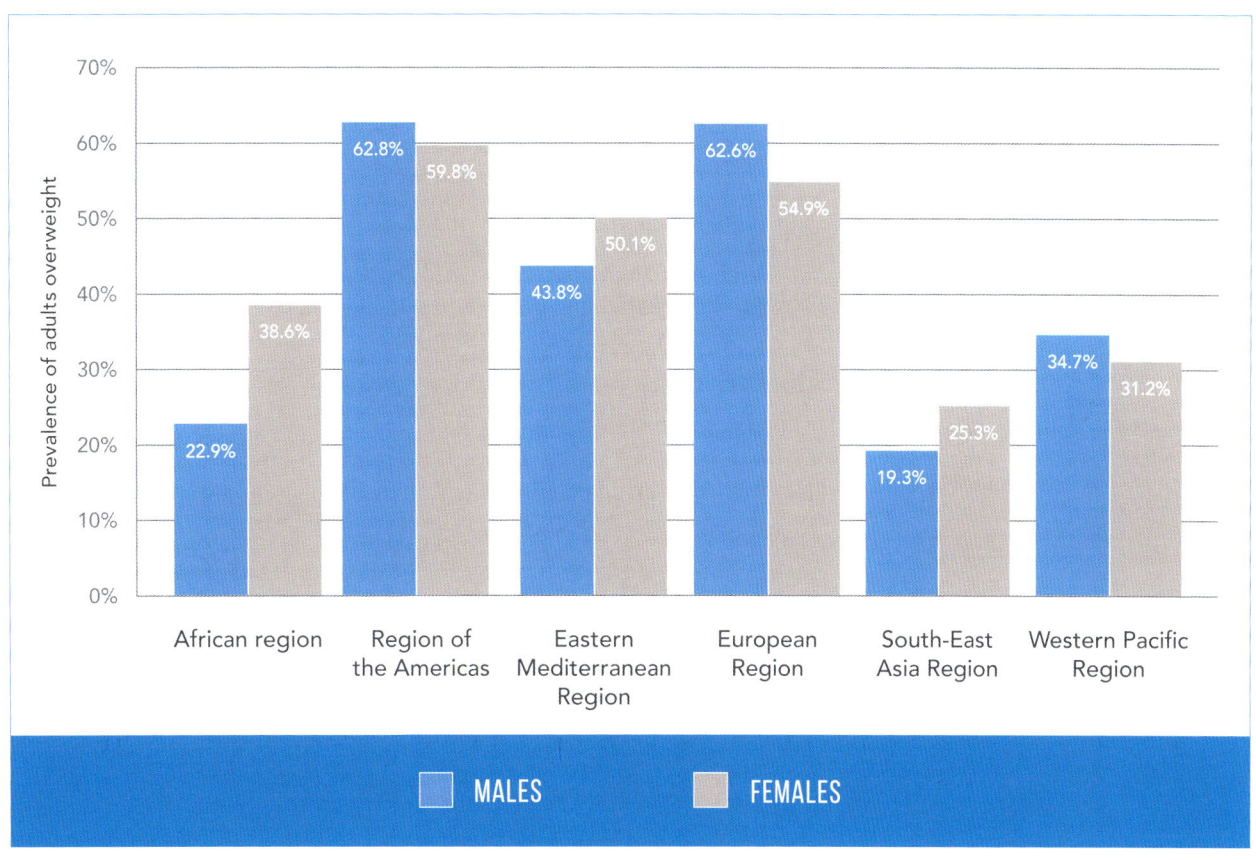

FIGURE 5B. PREVALENCE OF BEING OVERWEIGHT (BMI 25+) IN ADULTS OVER 18 YEARS, 2014, BY SEX AND COUNTRY INCOME GROUP

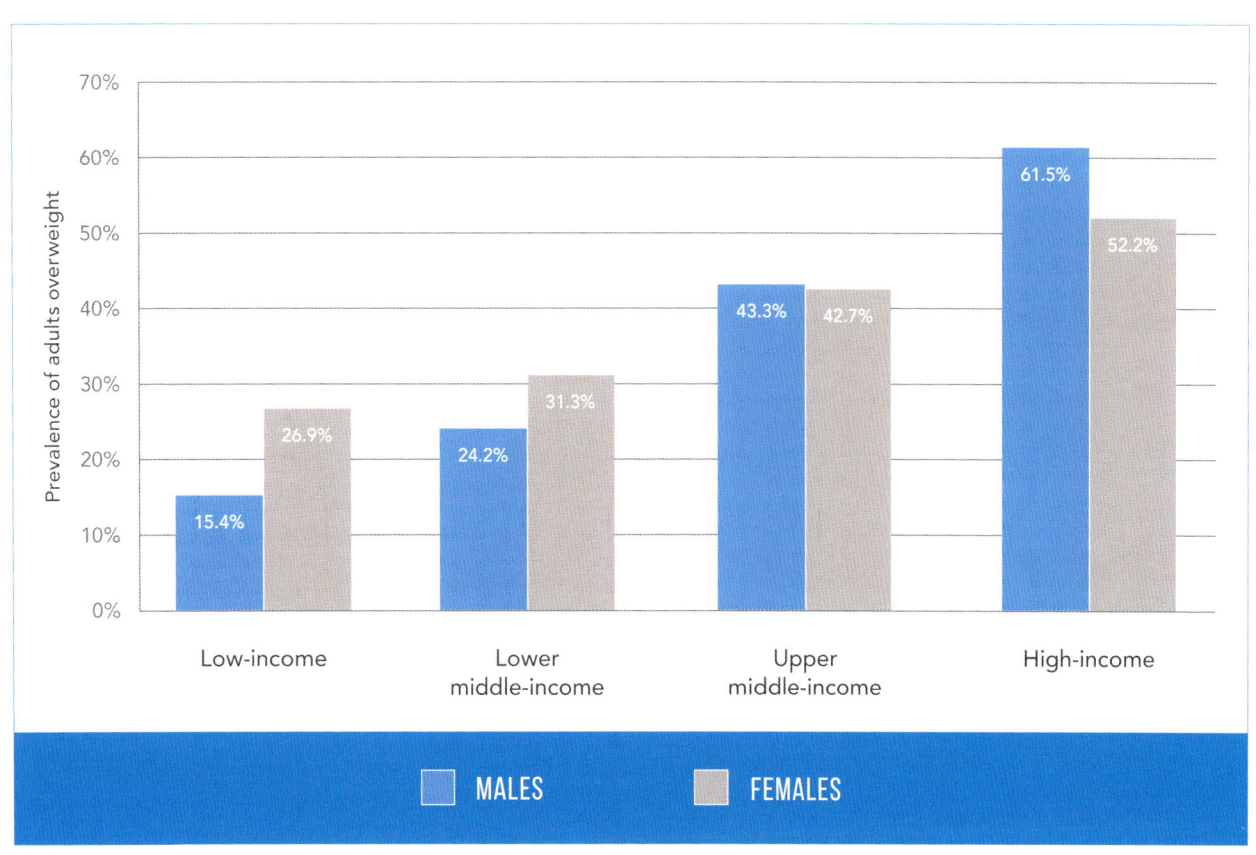

1.3 BURDEN AND TRENDS IN THE COMPLICATIONS OF DIABETES

Diabetes, if not well controlled, may cause blindness, kidney failure, lower limb amputation and several other long-term consequences that impact significantly on quality of life. There are no global estimates of diabetes-related end-stage renal disease, cardiovascular events, lower-extremity amputations or pregnancy complications, though these conditions affect many people living with diabetes. Where data are available – mostly from high-income countries – prevalence, incidence and trends vary hugely between countries *(18, 19)*.

LOSS OF VISION

Diabetic retinopathy caused 1.9% of moderate or severe visual impairment globally and 2.6% of blindness in 2010 *(20)*. Studies suggest that prevalence of any retinopathy in persons with diabetes is 35% while proliferative (vision-threatening) retinopathy is 7% *(21)*. However, retinopathy rates are higher among: people with type 1 diabetes; people with longer duration of diabetes; Caucasian populations; and possibly among people of lower socioeconomic status *(21)*.

END-STAGE RENAL DISEASE

Pooled data from 54 countries show that at least 80% of cases of end-stage renal disease (ESRD) are caused by diabetes, hypertension or a combination of the two *(18)*. The proportion of ESRD attributable to diabetes alone ranges from 12–55%. The incidence of ESRD is up to 10 times as high in adults with diabetes as those without. The prevalence of ESRD is heavily dependent on access to dialysis and renal replacement therapy – both of which are highly variable between (and in some cases within) countries.

CARDIOVASCULAR EVENTS

Adults with diabetes historically have a two or three times higher rate of cardiovascular disease (CVD) than adults without diabetes *(22)*. The risk of cardiovascular disease increases continuously with rising fasting plasma glucose levels, even before reaching levels sufficient for a diabetes diagnosis *(2, 3)*. The few countries in north America, Scandinavia and the United Kingdom of Great Britain and Northern Ireland that have studied time trends in the incidence of cardiovascular events (myocardial infarction, stroke or CVD mortality) report large reductions over the past 20 years among people with type 1 or type 2 diabetes *(23)*, although less than the reduction in the non-diabetic population. This decrease has been attributed to reduction in the prevalence of smoking and better management of diabetes and associated CVD risk factors.

LOWER EXTREMITY AMPUTATIONS

Diabetes appears to dramatically increase the risk of lower extremity amputation because of infected, non-healing foot ulcers *(19)*. Rates of amputation in populations with diagnosed diabetes are typically 10 to 20 times those of non-diabetic populations, and over the past decade have ranged from 1.5 to 3.5 events per 1000 persons per

> **Lower limb amputation rates are 10 to 20 times higher among people with diabetes**

year in populations with diagnosed diabetes. Encouragingly several studies show a 40% to 60% reduction in rates of amputations among adults with diabetes during the past 10–15 years in the United Kingdom, Sweden, Denmark, Spain, the United States of America and Australia *(19)*. No such data estimates exist for low- or middle-income countries.

1.4 SUMMARY

The number of people in the world with diabetes has quadrupled since 1980. Population growth and ageing have contributed to this increase, but are not solely responsible for it. The prevalence (age-standardized) of diabetes is growing in all regions. Global prevalence doubled from 1980 to 2014, mirroring a rise in overweight and obesity. Prevalence is growing most rapidly in low- and middle-income countries.

Blood glucose levels begin to have an impact on morbidity and mortality even below the diagnostic threshold for diabetes. Diabetes and higher-than-optimal blood glucose together are responsible for 3.7 million deaths, many of which could be prevented.

The numbers and trends presented in this section have implications for the health and well-being of populations, and for health systems. The complications of diabetes have significant impact on the individuals who experience them and their impact is also felt at population level. Diabetes is a serious threat to population health.

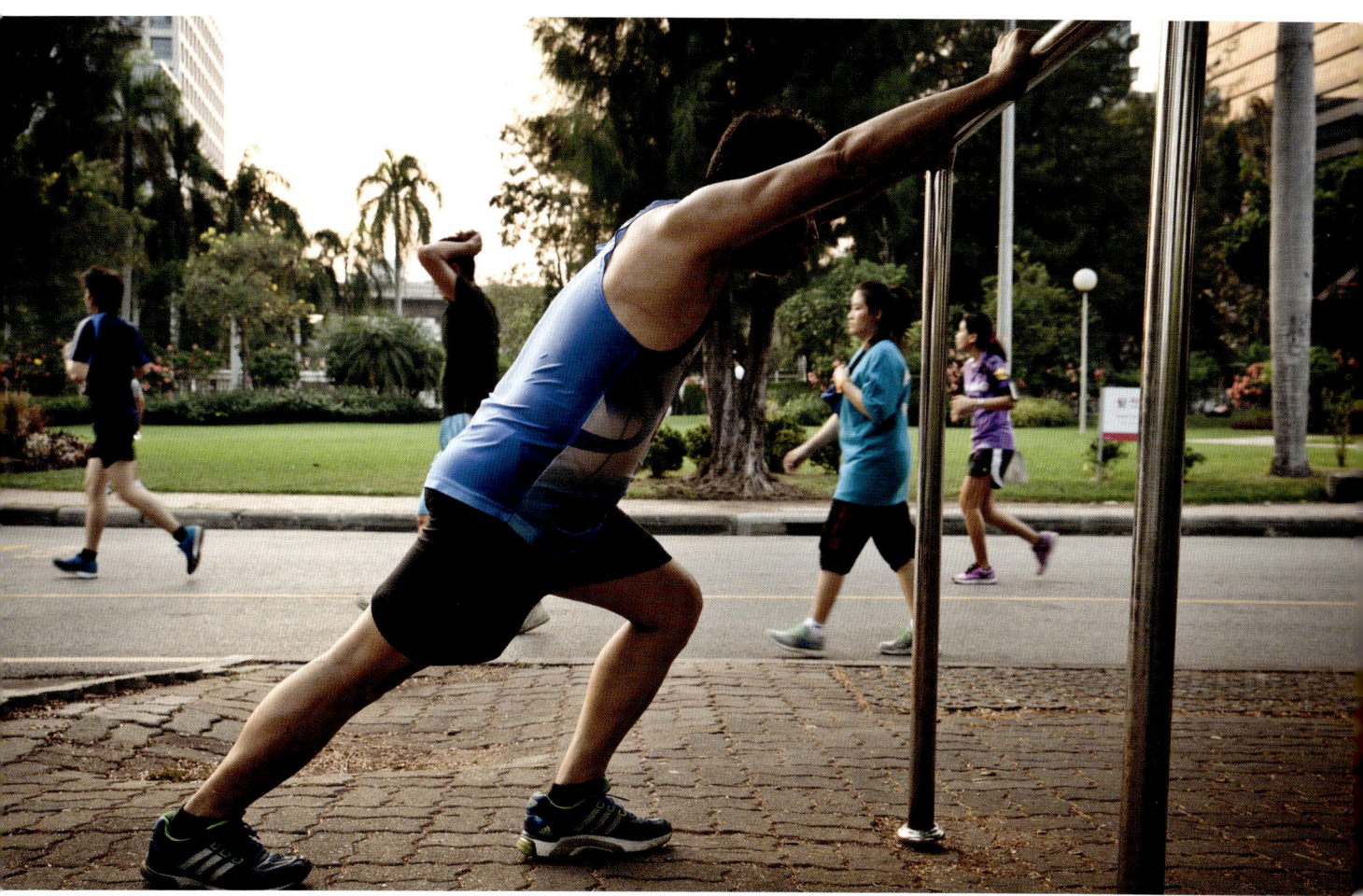

REFERENCES

1. WHO Mortality Database [online database]. Geneva: World Health Organization; (*http://apps.who.int/healthinfo/statistics/mortality/causeofdeath_query/*, accessed 12 January 2016).

2. Singh GM, Danaei G, Farzadfar F, Stevens GA, Woodward M, Wormser D et al. The age-specific quantitative effects of metabolic risk factors on cardiovascular diseases and diabetes: a pooled analysis. PLoS One 2013; 8(7):e65174.

3. Danaei G, Lawes CM, Vander HS, Murray CJ, Ezzati M. Global and regional mortality from ischaemic heart disease and stroke attributable to higher-than-optimum blood glucose concentration: comparative risk assessment. Lancet. 2006;368:(9548)1651–1659.

4. NCD Risk Factor Collaboration (NCD-RisC). Worldwide trends in diabetes since 1980: a pooled analysis of 751 population-based studies with 4*4 million participants. Lancet 2016; published online April 7. *http://dx.doi.org/10.1016/S0140-6736(16)00618-8*.

5. Incidence and trends of childhood type 1 diabetes worldwide, 1990–1999. Diabetes Medicine. 2006;23:(8)857–866.

6. Tuomilehto J. The emerging global epidemic of type 1 diabetes. Current Diabetes Reports. 2013;13:(6)795–804.

7. Patterson CC, Dahlquist GG, Gyurus E, Green A, Soltesz G. EURODIAB Study Group Incidence trends for childhood type 1 diabetes in Europe during 1989–2003 and predicted new cases 2005–20: a multicentre prospective registration study. Lancet. 2009;373:2027–2033.

8. Dabelea D. The accelerating epidemic of childhood diabetes. Lancet. 2009;373:(9680)1999–2000.

9. Gale EAM. The rise of childhood type 1 diabetes in the 20th century. Diabetes. 2002;51:3353–3361.

10. Diabetes: equity and social determinants. In Equity, social determinants and public health programmes. Blas E, Kuru A, eds. Geneva: World Health Organization; 2010.

11. Gakidou E, Mallinger L, Abbott-Klafter J, Guerrero R, Villalpando S, Ridaura RL, et al. Management of diabetes and associated cardiovascular risk factors in seven countries: a comparison of data from national health examination surveys. Bulletin of the World Health Organization. 2011);89:(3)172–183.

12. Tracking universal health coverage: first global monitoring report. Geneva: World Health Organization; 2015.

13. Beagley J, Guariguata L, Weil C, Motala AA. Global estimates of undiagnosed diabetes in adults. Diabetes Res Clin Pract. 2014;103: 150–160.

14. Jiwani A, Marseille E, Lohse N, Damm P, Hod M, Kahn JG. Gestational diabetes mellitus: results from a survey of country prevalence and practices. Journal of Maternal-Fetal Neonatal Medicine. 2012;25:(6)600–610.

15. Guariguata L, Linnenkamp U, Beagley J, Whiting DR, Cho NH. Global estimates of the prevalence of hyperglycaemia in pregnancy. Diabetes Res Clin Pract. 2014;103, (2) 176–185.

16. Global status report on noncommunicable diseases 2015. Geneva: World Health Organization; 2015.

17. Global action plan for the prevention and control of noncommunicable diseases 2013–2020. Geneva: World Health Organization; 2013.

18. United States Renal Data System. International Comparisons. In United States Renal Data System. 2014 USRDS annual data report: Epidemiology of kidney disease in the United States. Bethesda (MD): National Institutes of Health, National Institute of Diabetes and Digestive and Kidney Diseases; 2014:188–210.

19. Moxey PW, Gogalniceanu P, Hinchliffe RJ, Loftus IM, Jones KJ, Thompson MM, et al. Lower extremity amputations – a review of global variability in incidence. Diabetic Medicine. 2011;28:(10)1144–1153.

20. Bourne RR, Stevens GA, White RA, Smith JL, Flaxman SR, Price H, et al. Causes of vision loss worldwide, 1990–2010: a systematic analysis. Lancet Global Health. 2013;1:(6)e339-e349.

21. Yau JW, Rogers SL, Kawasaki R, Lamoureux EL, Kowalski JW, Bek T, et al. Global prevalence and major risk factors of diabetic retinopathy. Diabetes Care. 2012;35:(3)556–564.

22. Emerging Risk Factors Collaboration. Sarwar N, Gao P, Seshasai SR, Gobin R, Kaptoge S, Di Angelantonio E. Diabetes mellitus, fasting blood glucose concentration, and risk of vascular disease: a collaborative meta-analysis of 102 prospective studies. Lancet. 2010 Jun 26;375(9733):2215–22.

23. Barengo NC, Katoh S, Moltchanov V, Tajima N, Tuomilehto J. The diabetes-cardiovascular risk paradox: results from a Finnish population-based prospective study. European Heart Journal. 2008;29:(15)1889–1895.

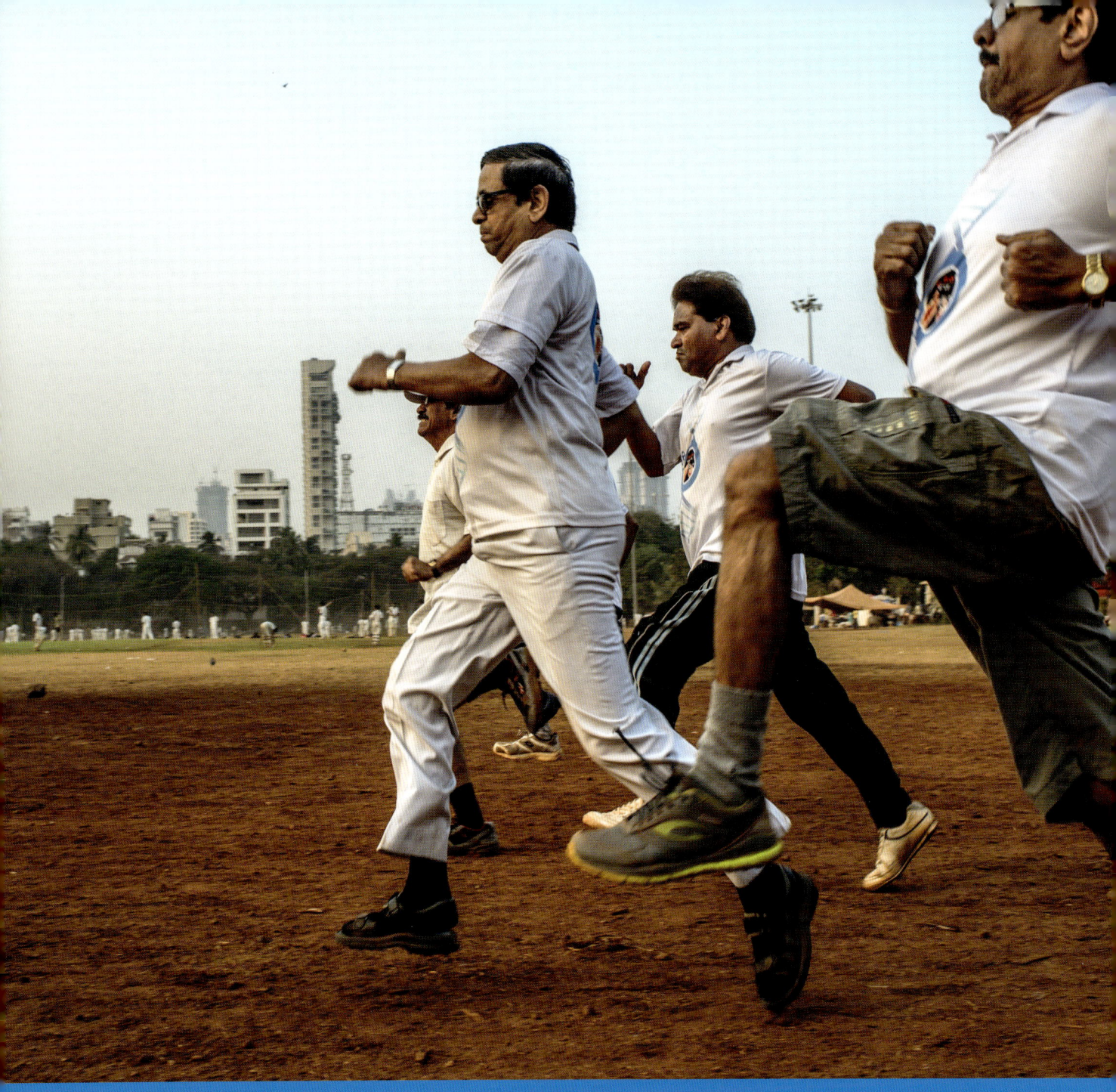

PART 2

PREVENTING DIABETES

KEY MESSAGES

Type 2 diabetes is largely preventable.

Multisectoral, population-based approaches are needed to reduce the prevalence of modifiable diabetes risk factors – such as overweight, obesity, physical inactivity and unhealthy diet – in the general population.

A combination of fiscal policies, legislation, changes to the environment and raising awareness of health risks works best for promoting healthier diets and physical activity.

Diabetes can be delayed or prevented in people who are overweight and have impaired glucose tolerance (IGT). Diet and physical activity interventions are more effective than medication.

The vast majority of the world's diabetes cases are type 2 *(1)*. Some risk factors for type 2 diabetes – such as genetics, ethnicity and age – are not modifiable. Others, such as being overweight or obese, unhealthy diet, insufficient physical activity and smoking are modifiable through behavioural and environmental changes. Several effective policy options are available to facilitate these behavioural changes and create supportive environments for healthy lifestyles. At the individual level, intensive interventions to improve diet and physical activity can prevent or delay the onset of type 2 diabetes in people at high risk.

2.1 POPULATION-BASED PREVENTION

There are strong indications – if not yet direct evidence – that population-based programmes aimed at modifiable risk factors can reduce the incidence of diabetes while also lowering blood pressure and other cardiovascular risk factors. Population-based data from Cuba show a fall in type 2 diabetes during a period of economic crisis when the population experienced a reduction in calorie intake and a simultaneous increase in physical activity *(2)*, suggesting population-wide changes in diet and physical activity do affect type 2 diabetes prevalence.

Actions to address overweight and obesity are critical to preventing type 2 diabetes. Evidence on what works as a package of interventions for the prevention of overweight and obesity is limited, but much is known about promotion of healthy diet and physical activity, which are key to prevention and attaining the global obesity and diabetes target (see Box 1, page 16). Promoting healthy diets and increasing physical activity in the population will help reduce the occurrence of obesity and type 2 diabetes, and will accrue additional benefits by reducing complications among people with all types of diabetes and glucose intolerance. WHO's recommendations for healthy diet and physical activity relevant to diabetes are summarized in Box 2.

Population-level interventions to reduce tobacco use may contribute to prevention of type 2 diabetes, given emerging evidence of a link between smoking and type 2 diabetes risk. Active tobacco use can be reduced through a set of legislative, regulatory, fiscal and educational measures including graphic warnings on cigarette packs, bans on advertising and promotion, raising taxes on tobacco and implementing mass media campaigns (6). WHO Member States have committed to these and other actions through WHO's Framework Convention on Tobacco Control, which entered into force in 2005. Reducing population exposure to tobacco may also reduce diabetes-related complications, in part through reducing cardiovascular risk.

BOX 2. HEALTHY DIET AND PHYSICAL ACTIVITY

Adults can reduce their risk of type 2 diabetes and improve insulin sensitivity and glucose uptake through regular and adequate levels of physical activity and healthy diets that include sufficient consumption of dietary fibre, and replacing saturated fatty acids with polyunsaturated fatty acids. WHO has developed recommendations on healthy diet and physical activity that, if implemented, can reduce an individual's risk of type 2 diabetes and other NCDs.

Dietary recommendations by WHO and the Food and Agriculture Organization (FAO) for the prevention of type 2 diabetes include limiting saturated fatty acid intake to less than 10% of total energy intake (and for high risk groups, less than 7%); and achieving adequate intakes of dietary fibre (minimum daily intake of 20 g) through regular consumption of wholegrain cereals, legumes, fruits and vegetables (3). WHO is currently updating its guidelines on fat intake and carbohydrate intake, which will include recommendations on dietary fibre as well as fruits and vegetables. WHO strongly recommends reducing the intake of free sugars to less than 10% of total energy intake and suggests that further reduction to 5% could have additional health benefits (4).

WHO recommendations on physical activity are provided for different age groups (5):

- It is recommended that children and youth aged 5–17 years should do at least 60 minutes of moderate- to vigorous-intensity physical activity daily.

- It is recommended that adults aged 18–64 years should do at least 150 minutes of moderate-intensity aerobic physical activity (for example brisk walking, jogging, gardening) spread throughout the week, or at least 75 minutes of vigorous-intensity aerobic physical activity throughout the week, or an equivalent combination of moderate- and vigorous-intensity activity.

- For older adults the same amount of physical activity is recommended, but should also include balance and muscle strengthening activity tailored to their ability and circumstances.

The rise in diabetes risk factors has occurred in the context of changes in the social, economic and physical environments in which we are born and live. Population-based prevention aims not only to reduce risk factors for diabetes and NCDs, but also to shape the broader environments in which people live, eat, study, work and play, so that healthy choices are accessible and easy to make.

No single policy or intervention can achieve changes of this magnitude. Such an agenda calls for a "whole-of-government" approach, in which all sectors systematically consider the health impact of policies in trade, agriculture, finance, transport, education and urban planning – recognizing that health is enhanced or obstructed as a result of policies in these and other areas.

A LIFE-COURSE APPROACH TO PREVENTING DIABETES

Taking a life-course perspective is essential for type 2 diabetes prevention. Early in life, when eating and physical activity habits are formed and when the long-term regulation of energy balance may be programmed *(7)*, there is a critical window for intervention to mitigate the risk of obesity and type 2 diabetes later in life *(8)*. The report of the WHO Commission on Ending Childhood Obesity *(9)* provides a comprehensive, integrated package of recommendations to address childhood obesity that will contribute to the reduction of risks for developing type 2 diabetes. A life-course approach to diabetes would also recognize the increasing risk that comes with advancing age, and the need to identify the unique needs for risk reduction in older adults.

IMPROVING EARLY CHILDHOOD NUTRITION

Strategies to improve early childhood nutrition should not be overlooked among type 2 diabetes prevention efforts. These actions must be aimed at improving maternal health and nutritional status and infant and young child-feeding practices, focusing on the first 1000 days from a woman's pregnancy to her child's second birthday *(3)*. Specific measures include promoting the nutritional well-being of pregnant women; promotion of breastfeeding, including the implementation of the Code of Marketing of Breast Milk Substitutes; improving the nutritional status of infants and young children through exclusive breastfeeding up to 6 months of age; introducing a variety of safe, nutritious and adequate foods at 6 months of age to complement breastfeeding (which should continue until babies are 2 years of age or more); promoting growth in height; preventing the consumption of foods that are high in energy, fats, sugars and sodium; and facilitating physical activity *(10)*.

SUPPORTIVE ENVIRONMENTS FOR PHYSICAL ACTIVITY

The physical or built environment plays an important role in facilitating physical activity for many people. Urban planning and active transport policies can ensure that walking, cycling and other forms of non-motorized

> **Actions to address overweight and obesity are critical to preventing type 2 diabetes**

Policies that increase the price of foods high in fat, sugar and salt can decrease their consumption

transport are accessible and safe for all. The physical environment can also provide sports, recreation and leisure facilities, and ensure there are adequate safe spaces for active living for both children and adults *(11)*. The poorest groups in society, especially women, may have less time and fewer resources to participate in leisure-time activity, making policy interventions that target active transport and incidental physical activity throughout the day much more important. Promotion of stair use – including placement of physical activity promotion messages on stairs – as part of a workplace programme has been shown to increase awareness and use of stairs *(12)*.

The sports sector can encourage regular structured activities, especially among children and adolescents, and can strengthen the link between physical activity, sports and health. Partnerships with communities, the private sector and nongovernmental organizations can also contribute to developing facilities for physical activity.

SETTINGS-BASED INTERVENTIONS

Settings-based interventions can support diabetes prevention and control. These interventions reach families and communities where they live, study, work and play to implement both population-wide and individual high-risk interventions. Settings-based interventions should be comprehensive, make use of existing programmes when possible and focus on actions that do not require additional resources.

A whole-of-school approach that focuses on improving both diet and physical activity can be very effective in improving dietary patterns both inside and outside school *(13)*. Successful school-based physical activity interventions should result in consistent improvements in the knowledge, attitudes and behaviour of children and, when tested, in physical and clinical outcomes *(14)*. WHO's health-promoting schools initiative has demonstrated the importance of highlighting both the impact on attendance and educational achievement, as well as the health benefits of a whole-of-school approach *(15)*.

Workplace interventions addressing diet and physical activity can be effective in changing behaviours and health-related outcomes *(16)*. Healthy-eating messages in cafés and restaurants have been shown to stimulate consumption of healthy food – provided that healthy food items are made available as part of the intervention *(17)*. Workplaces can help develop environments that are conducive to physical activity at work and provide incentives and opportunities for active commuting to and from work. Workplaces may offer their employees free or discounted vouchers for physical activity facilities.

FISCAL, LEGISLATIVE AND REGULATORY MEASURES FOR HEALTHY DIET

Fiscal measures. Price is often reported as a barrier to people buying and consuming healthy foods. Likewise, policy action to increase the price of foods high in fat, sugar and salt can decrease their consumption (see Box 3). There is emerging evidence that appropriately designed fiscal policies, when implemented together with other policy actions, have the potential to promote healthier diets *(18)*. Fiscal policies should be considered a key component of a comprehensive strategy for prevention and control of NCDs, including diabetes.

Trade and agricultural policies that promote healthy diets. Trade measures have proven effective in reducing the availability of unhealthy foods and changing people's diet. For example, in 2000 Fiji banned the supply of high-fat mutton flaps under the Trading Standards Act. Also, in Mauritius, the reduction of saturated fatty acids in cooking oil and their replacement with soya bean oil is estimated to have changed consumption patterns for the best, and reduced average total cholesterol levels *(19)*. Changes in agricultural subsidies to encourage fruit and vegetable production can be beneficial in increasing their consumption and improving diet. Evidence strongly supports the use of such subsidies and related policies to facilitate sustained long-term production, transport and marketing of healthier foods *(20)*.

Regulation of marketing of foods high in sugars, fats and salt. There is ample evidence that the marketing of foods and non-alcoholic beverages influences children's knowledge, attitudes, beliefs and preferences. WHO has developed a set of recommendations and an implementation framework on the marketing of foods and non-alcoholic beverages to children *(26)*. This aims to assist Member States in designing and implementing new policies – or strengthening existing ones – that regulate the marketing of food to children.

Nutrition labelling is a regulatory tool that can guide consumers towards healthier food choices.

BOX 3. THE "SUGAR-SWEETENED BEVERAGE TAX", MEXICO

The prevalence of overweight and obesity in Mexico stands at more than 33% in children and around 70% in adults *(21)*. Mexico has the highest prevalence of diabetes among Organization for Economic Cooperation and Development (OECD) member countries *(22)*, and the highest per capita consumption of soft drinks worldwide *(23)*.

In January 2014 Mexico implemented a nationwide tax on drinks containing added sugar (bebidas azucaradas) that increased their price by over 10%. While it is too early to draw far-reaching conclusions, one analysis estimated that the 10% increase in the price of added-sugar drinks was associated with an 11.6% decrease in the quantity consumed *(24)*.

During the first year of the tax, purchases of taxed sugar-sweetened beverages decreased by an average of 6% compared to what would have been expected without implementation of the tax (25), with higher reductions found in households of low socioeconomic status.

Interventions that promote healthy diet, physical activity and weight loss can prevent type 2 diabetes in people at high risk

Nutrition labelling comprises nutrient declarations and supplementary nutrition information commonly referred to as front-of-pack labelling. The nutrient declarations provide quantitative information and usually appear on small print on the back of packages; front-of-pack labelling is designed to assist in interpreting nutrient declarations. Front-of-pack labelling may also encourage manufacturers to make the composition of retail food products healthier, to achieve competitive advantages or to avoid unfavourable disclosures about food composition. There is evidence that simple, front-of-pack labels on packaged foods, or point-of-purchase information in grocery stores, cafés or restaurants, can be beneficial to support healthier options, as can menu labelling *(27)*.

EDUCATION, SOCIAL MARKETING AND MOBILIZATION

Consumer awareness and knowledge of healthy diet and physical activity can be achieved through sustained media and educational campaigns aimed at increasing consumption of healthy foods (or reducing consumption of less healthy ones), and increasing physical activity. These campaigns have greater impact and are more cost-effective when used within multicomponent strategies *(28)*. For example, a social marketing campaign in Tonga using netball to promote physical activity among women as part of a national NCD campaign has resulted in increased participation both in netball and leisure-time physical activity by women *(29)*.

2.2 PREVENTING DIABETES IN PEOPLE AT HIGH RISK

Research in different parts of the world has shown that intensive interventions that change people's diet, increase physical activity and lead to the loss of excess body weight can prevent type 2 diabetes in people with impaired glucose tolerance, with or without impaired fasting glucose. For example, the Diabetes Prevention Program (DPP) in the USA *(30)*, the Finnish Diabetes Prevention Study (DPS) *(31)* and the Chinese Da Qing Study showed that active intervention, lasting 2 to 6 years, could have extended benefits for glycaemic and cardiovascular outcomes that last for 10 to 20 years *(32)*.

Several pharmacological interventions (for example, metformin and acarbose) have also been shown to prevent or delay type 2 diabetes but, in the majority of studies, this is not as effective as changes in diet and physical activity, and the effect dissipates after discontinuation of the medication *(33, 34)*.

Knowledge gained from these proof-of-concept studies confirms that type 2 diabetes can be delayed or prevented, but turning this knowledge into large-scale impact brings significant challenges. The success of these programmes depends on the feasibility of identifying, assessing and successfully involving high-risk groups (see Box 4). Careful decisions are required about how to assess diabetes risk, how to support those identified as high-risk, and how to ensure care for those diagnosed with diabetes as a result of the risk assessment. The individual or high-risk

> **BOX 4. EXAMPLES OF TOOLS TO ASSESS THE RISK OF HAVING CURRENT OR FUTURE DIABETES**
>
> Measurement of blood glucose remains the best predictor of type 2 diabetes risk, though a wide and ever-increasing range of biomarkers has been reported to predict future development of type 2 diabetes. The risk of having or developing type 2 diabetes can also be assessed using tools that cover variables such as age, sex, history of GDM and family history of diabetes, as well as clinical measures of body mass index, waist circumference and waist-hip ratio. Several tools that assess the risk of having undiagnosed or future diabetes have been developed and adapted for use in diverse populations:
>
> - FINRISK: a simple score adapted for use in several countries, using age, BMI, waist circumference, history of anti-hypertensive drug treatment and high blood glucose, physical activity, and daily consumption of fruits, berries or vegetables to estimate risk *(35)*.
>
> - AUSDRISK: a 10-item questionnaire that estimates risk of progression to type 2 diabetes over 5 years. Its scoring includes questions based on age, sex, ethnicity, family history of diabetes, history of abnormal glucose metabolism, smoking status, current hypertensive treatment, physical activity, fruit and vegetable consumption, and waist circumference *(36)*.
>
> - IDRS (Indian Diabetes Risk Score): a simplified risk score for identifying undiagnosed diabetic subjects using four simple parameters – age, waist circumference, family history of diabetes and physical activity. IDRS is an inexpensive and simple tool for screening for risk of undiagnosed diabetes *(37)*.

approach needs to be translated into well-defined strategies for implementation at community level and in national programmes, in accordance with available resources. It has the potential to overwhelm primary care services, where the responsibility for intervention usually lies.

There is no universal answer regarding the advisability of population screening for type 2 diabetes risk. Assessment of diabetes risk should not be confused with the total risk approach to cardiovascular disease risk in which diabetes is included as one component. Diabetes is not only a risk factor for CVD, it also has its own specific complications. However, given the overlap of diabetes and CVD risk factors, combined screening for risk of both conditions is a rational approach. The decision to systematically look for people at high risk of diabetes and CVD is a strategic one specific to each health-care setting, and will depend, at least in part, on the numbers likely to be identified and the resources available to adequately deal with them (see also Chapter 4 for early detection of undiagnosed diabetes).

Whether or not intensive individual interventions are made available, and whether or not systematic assessment of risk is undertaken, primary health-care services must be equipped to manage people with high risk of type 2 diabetes. Clinical vigilance alone, even in the absence of systems for early detection of type 2 diabetes or systematic risk prediction, will identify people who are at high

Much type 2 diabetes results from risk factors that can be reduced using a combination of approaches at population and individual levels.

risk for future development of type 2 diabetes. These people should receive (as a minimum) repeat counselling on weight loss, diet, physical activity and smoking.

While type 2 diabetes is potentially preventable, the causes and risk factors for type 1 diabetes remain unknown and prevention strategies have not yet been successful (see Box 5).

2.3 SUMMARY

Much type 2 diabetes results from modifiable risk factors that can be reduced using a combination of approaches at population and individual levels. Creating supportive policy, social and physical environments for healthy lifestyles is a key aspect of type 2 diabetes prevention. Sustaining the lifestyle changes needed to reduce risk requires supportive family and social networks, as well as an enabling food system and physical environment. Healthy food and opportunities for physical activity must be available and affordable.

BOX 5. TOWARDS PREVENTION OF TYPE 1 DIABETES

A variety of immunological approaches have been successful at preventing a disease similar to human type 1 diabetes in laboratory animals. As a result, hope has emerged that analogous interventions in humans might prevent type 1 diabetes or significantly slow the decline in beta cell function that characterizes the condition. Effective intervention of this nature could significantly reduce the incidence of type 1 diabetes and its long-term complications, greatly enhancing quality of life for people living with it.

Primary prevention trials involving dietary modification have been conducted with infants identified through genetic screening as being at highest risk of developing type 1 diabetes. Tested interventions and factors have included early exposure to cows' milk; the age of introduction of solid foods; supplementation with an omega-3 fatty acid; and supplementation with vitamin D. None of the trials has shown a reduction in type 1 incidence.

Other trials have focused on relatives of people with type 1 diabetes. Two large randomized clinical trials have explored the use of vitamin B6 supplementation in adults and children who are related to people with type 1 diabetes and are pancreatic islet antibody-positive, with negative results. Injected insulin and oral insulin have also been explored as preventive interventions in children with antibodies to insulin. The overall results were negative but a subgroup with the highest concentration of anti-insulin antibodies at the start of the trial showed some delay in onset.

Other approaches, as yet unsuccessful, have been treatment of people at high risk with nasal insulin, low-dose cyclosporine and with a monoclonal antibody.

Source: (38)

The WHO Global NCD Action Plan 2013–2020 sets out policy options for reducing modifiable NCD risk factors. Scaled-up implementation of these should reduce the occurrence of type 2 diabetes. Achieving the global voluntary target to halt the rising trend of obesity and diabetes will, however, require innovation and the scaling-up in particular of interventions to promote healthy diets and physical activity, as well as innovative ways to measure impact and expand the evidence base for population-wide prevention.

Implementation of effective strategies to reduce modifiable risk factors for diabetes and other NCDs frequently face powerful industry opposition. Trade measures and regulatory policies such as taxes on foods and beverages; restriction of marketing of unhealthy foods and non-alcoholic beverages; and implementing effective front-of-package labelling frequently face opposition from industry. Interference by food and beverage companies in policy-making and conflicts of interest can lead to the adoption of industry self-regulatory schemes that tend to be less effective than government regulation.

A whole-of-government approach, and even a whole-of-society approach, is essential to the success of most of these strategies. Without support from the highest level of government, it may be difficult to engage effectively with other key sectors, such as trade, industry, agriculture and education.

As noted by the WHO Commission on Ending Childhood Obesity, a comprehensive approach is needed to change the environmental factors that encourage weight gain and obesity (9). Action is required both to increase physical activity and healthy diet, and to reduce sedentary behaviours and intake of unhealthy foods and beverages. Particular consideration should be given to the impact of these interventions on populations of lower socioeconomic status, who often lack access to healthier foods and opportunities for physical activity.

REFERENCES

1. Definition, diagnosis and classification of diabetes mellitus and its complications. Part 1: Diagnosis and classification of diabetes mellitus. WHO/NCD/NCS/99.2. Geneva: World Health Organization; 1999.

2. Franco M, Bilal U, Orduñez P, Benet M, Morejon A, Caballero B et al. Population-wide weight loss and regain in relation to diabetes burden and cardiovascular mortality in Cuba 1980-2010: repeated cross sectional surveys and ecological comparison of secular trends. British Medical Journal. 2013;346.

3. Diet, nutrition and the prevention of chronic diseases. Report of a joint WHO/FAO expert consultation. WHO Technical Report series No 916. Geneva: World Health Organization; 2003.

4. Sugars intake for adults and children. Guidelines. Geneva: World Health Organization; 2015.

5. Global recommendations on physical activity for health. Geneva: World Health Organization; 2010.

6. Tobacco. WHO Fact Sheet No 339. Geneva: World Health Organization; 2015.

7. Vickers MH. Early life nutrition, epigenetics and programming of later life disease. Nutrients. 2014;6:(6)2165–2178.

8. Global nutrition targets 2025: Childhood overweight [policy brief]. Geneva: World Health Organization; 2014.

9. Commission on Ending Childhood Obesity. Geneva: World Health Organization; 2015.

10. Darnton-Hill I, Nishida C, James WP. A life course approach to diet, nutrition and the prevention of chronic diseases. Public Health Nutrition. 2004;7:(1A)101–121.

11. Mozaffarian D, Afshin A, Benowitz NL, Bittner V, Daniels SR, Franch HA. Population approaches to improve diet, physical activity, and smoking habits: a scientific statement from the American Heart Association. Circulation. 2012;126:(12)1514–1563.

12. Interventions on diet and physical activity. What works. Geneva: World Health Organization; 2009.

13. School policy framework: implementation of the WHO global strategy on diet, physical activity and health. Geneva: World Health Organization; 2008.

14. Kahn EB, Ramsey LT, Brownson RC, Heath GW, Howze EH, Powell KE, et al. The effectiveness of interventions to increase physical activity. A systematic review. American Journal of Preventive Medicine. 2002;22:(4 Suppl)73–107.

15. Health-promoting schools. A healthy setting for living, learning and working. Geneva: World Health Organization; 1998.

16. Task Force on Community Preventive Services. A recommendation to improve employee weight status through worksite health promotion programs targeting nutrition, physical activity or both. American Journal of Preventive Medicine. 2009;37:358–359.

17. Preventing noncommunicable diseases in the workplace through diet and physical activity. WHO/World Economic Forum report of a joint event. Geneva: World Health Organization/World Economic Forum; 2008.

18. Fiscal policy options with potential for improving diets for the prevention of noncommunicable diseases (NCDs). Geneva: World Health Organization; 2015.

19. Uusitalo U, Feskens EJ, Tuomilehto J, Dowse G, Haw U, Fareed D, et al. Fall in total cholesterol concentration over 5 years in association with changes in fatty acid composition of cooking oil in Mauritius: cross sectional survey. British Medical Journal. 1996;313:(7064)1044–1046.

20. Wallinga D. Agricultural policy and childhood obesity: a food systems and public health commentary. Health Affairs (Millwood). 2010;29:(3)405–410.

21. Gutierrez J, River-Dommarco J, Shamah-Levy T, et al. Encuesta Nacional de Salud y Nutricion 2012. Resultados Nacionales [National Health and Nutrition Survey, 2012. National Results]. Mexico: National Institute of Public Health; 2012.

22. Organization of Economic Cooperation and Development. Health at a Glance 2015. Washington DC: Brookings Institution Press; 2015.

23. EuroMonitor International. Passport Global Market Information Database [*http://www.euromonitor.com/passport*]

24. Colchero MA, Salgado JC, Unar-Munguia M, Hernandez-Avila M, Rivera-Dommarco JA. Price elasticity of the demand for sugar-sweetened beverages and soft drinks in Mexico. Economics and Human Biology. 2015;19:129–137.

25. Colchero MA, Popkin BM, Rivera JA, Ng SW. Beverage purchases from stores in Mexico under the excise tax on sugar sweetened beverages: observational study. British Medical Journal. 2016;352:h6704.

26. Set of recommendations on the marketing of foods and non-alcoholic beverages to children. Geneva: World Health Organization; 2010.

27. Kelly B. Front-of-pack labelling: a comprehensive review. Geneva: World Health Organization (in press).

28. Cecchini M, Sassi F, Lauer JA, Lee YY, Guajardo-Barron V, Chisholm D. Tackling of unhealthy diets, physical inactivity, and obesity: health effects and cost-effectiveness. Lancet. 2010;376:(9754)1775–1784.

29. Turk T, Latu N, Cocker-Palu E, Liavaa V, Vivili P, Gloede S, et al. Using rapid assessment and response to operationalise physical activity strategic health communication campaigns in Tonga. Health Promotion Journal of Australia. 2013;24:(1)13–19.

30. Knowler WC, Barrett-Connor E, Fowler SE, Hamman RF, Lachin JM, Walker EA, et al. Reduction in the incidence of type 2 diabetes with lifestyle intervention or metformin. New England Journal of Medicine. 2002;346:(6)393–403.

31. Uusitupa M, Peltonen M, Lindstrom J, Aunola S, Ilanne-Parikka P, Keinanen-Kiukaanniemi, et al. Ten-year mortality and cardiovascular morbidity in the Finnish Diabetes Prevention Study – secondary analysis of the randomized trial. PLoS.One. 2009;4:(5)e5656.

32. Li G, Zhang P, Wang J, Gregg EW, Yang W, Gong Q, et al. The long-term effect of lifestyle interventions to prevent diabetes in the China Da Qing Diabetes Prevention Study: a 20-year follow-up study. Lancet. 2008;371:(9626)1783–1789.

33. Merlotti C, Morabito A, Pontiroli AE. Prevention of type 2 diabetes; a systematic review and meta-analysis of different intervention strategies. Diabetes, Obesity and Metabolism. 2014;16:(8)719–727.

34. Orozco LJ, Buchleitner AM, Gimenez-Perez G, Roque IF, Richter B, Mauricio D. Exercise or exercise and diet for preventing type 2 diabetes mellitus. Cochrane Database of Systematic Reviews. 2008;(3):CD003054.

35. Lindstrom J, Tuomilehto J. The diabetes risk score: a practical tool to predict type 2 diabetes risk. Diabetes Care. 2003;26:(3)725–731.

36. Chen L, Magliano DJ, Balkau B, Colagiuri S, Zimmet PZ, Tonkin AM, et al. AUSDRISK: an Australian type 2 diabetes risk assessment tool based on demographic, lifestyle and simple anthropometric measures. Medical Journal of Australia. 2010;192:(4)197–202.

37. Mohan V, Sandeep S, Deepa M, Gokulakrishnan K, Datta M, Deepa R. A diabetes risk score helps identify metabolic syndrome and cardiovascular risk in Indians – the Chennai Urban Rural Epidemiology Study (CURES-38). Diabetes, Obesity and Metabolism. 2007;9:(3)337–343.

38. Skyler JS. in International textbook on diabetes mellitus, 4 ed. Chichester, UK; Wiley Blackwell, 2015, pp. 541–549.

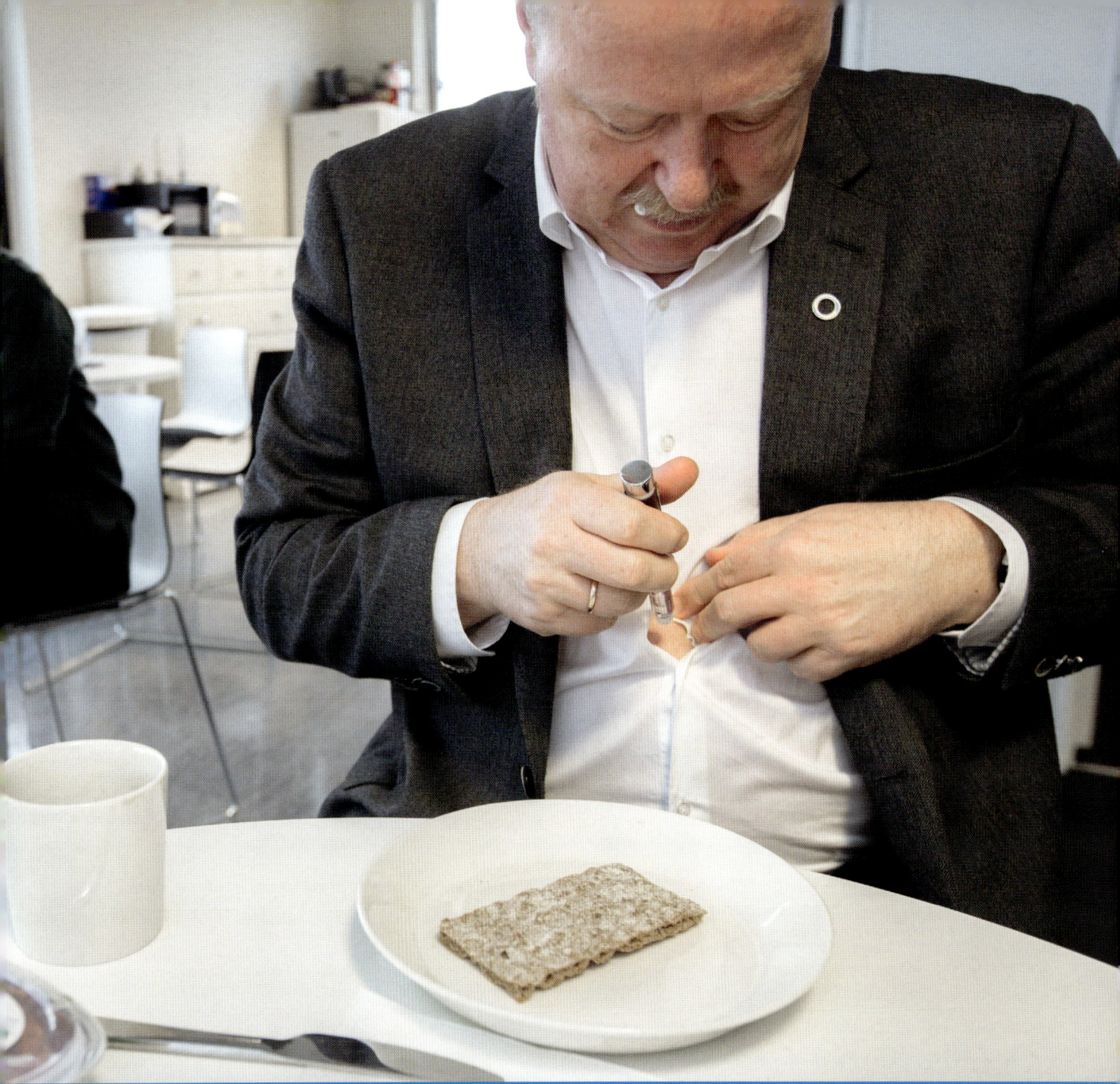

PART 3

MANAGING DIABETES

KEY MESSAGES

People with diabetes can live long and healthy lives if their diabetes is detected and well-managed.

Good management using a standardized protocol can potentially prevent complications and premature death from diabetes using: a small set of generic medicines; interventions to promote healthy lifestyles; patient education to facilitate self-care; regular screening for early detection and treatment of complications through a multidisciplinary team.

Facilities for diabetes diagnosis and management should be available in primary health-care settings, with an established referral and back-referral system.

In countries with a high burden of diabetes and tuberculosis or HIV/AIDS, there is frequent coexistence of these conditions and integrated management is recommended.

Access to essential medicines (including life-saving insulin) and technologies is worryingly limited in low- and middle-income countries.

Well-structured health services can provide the key interventions and regular follow-up necessary to help people with diabetes live long and relatively healthy lives, even though it is a chronic, progressive disease. Many of these interventions are known to be cost-effective or cost-saving, and are feasible even in low-resource settings (1, 2, 3). Controlling blood glucose levels and cardiovascular disease risk through counselling to promote a healthy diet and physical activity, and through use of medicines, is considered a "best buy" for reducing the health impact of NCDs.

Encouragingly, reductions in the rates of several diabetes-related complications (amputation, cardiovascular disease, vision loss, end-stage renal disease) have been observed in countries that have adequate data to examine trends over time (4). Where reductions in complications have been observed at population level they are likely to be the result of improvements in the management of key risk factors such as smoking, blood pressure and lipid levels, and blood glucose, along with improvements in the organization and quality of care.

3.1 DIAGNOSIS AND EARLY DETECTION

The starting point for living well with diabetes is an early diagnosis – the longer a person lives with undiagnosed and untreated diabetes, the worse the health outcomes are likely to be. Easy

> **The longer a person lives with undiagnosed and untreated diabetes, the worse their health outcomes are likely to be**

access to basic diagnostics for diabetes is therefore essential and diagnosis should be available in primary health-care settings.

Type 1 diabetes often presents with symptoms that prompt the patient to contact health services – thirst, weight loss and copious urination. Type 2 diabetes often shows no symptoms, and some patients contact health services because of a complication such as vision loss, heart attack or limb gangrene. Type 2 diabetes develops slowly and there is often a very long period of time in which the disease is present but undetected.

Diabetes is diagnosed by measuring glucose in a blood sample taken while the patient is in a fasting state, or 2 hours after a 75 g oral load of glucose has been taken (see Annex A). Diabetes can also be diagnosed by measuring glycated haemoglobin (HbA1c), even if the patient is not in a fasting state (5). HbA1c reflects the average blood glucose concentration over the past few weeks, rather than the blood glucose concentration at that moment (reflected by the fasting and 2-hour blood glucose measurements mentioned above). However, the test is more costly than blood glucose measurement (5).

Blood glucose measurement to diagnose diabetes should be available at the primary health-care level. If laboratory analysis of venous plasma glucose is not feasible, point-of-care devices that measure glucose in capillary blood and meet current International Standardization Organization (ISO) standards are an acceptable alternative. Unfortunately, testing devices and supplies are often not available where or when necessary – one survey found the availability of blood glucose meters ranged from 21% to 100% in facilities visited in five developing countries (6).

EARLY DETECTION OF TYPE 2 DIABETES

Whether people should be screened or not for type 2 diabetes is a much-debated question and currently there is no definitive evidence from randomized trials to answer it. Some evidence suggests there are benefits to early detection and treatment, largely because the reduced lead time between onset and diagnosis speeds the treatment of cardiovascular risk factors – particularly improved management of lipids and blood pressure (7).

The decision to put in place (or not put in place) systems for early detection is a strategic one that depends on a number of factors. Screening programmes will increase the number of clinically diagnosed cases of type 2 diabetes and as such will increase the health-care system workload, not only in dealing with the process of early detection but, more importantly, in dealing with the increased number of clinically diagnosed cases that will be found (8). No system should be established without consideration of whether local health-care resources are sufficient to cope with this extra workload. Simply adding new cases to a health-care system without additional investment will, in the absence of compensating efficiencies, result in poorer average care (9).

> **BOX 6. PEN FA'A, SAMOA: ISLAND FAMILIES COME TOGETHER TO COMBAT NCDs, IMPROVE HEALTH AND SAVE LIVES**
>
> Half of all adults in Samoa are at high risk of developing NCDs such as cancer, diabetes and heart disease. Despite improvements in overall health over the past few decades, the island has a high and growing prevalence of NCDs.
>
> In response to this public health threat, PEN Fa'a Samoa (an adaptation of WHO PEN protocols), with support from WHO, was initiated in November 2014 in several demonstration sites. PEN Fa'a Samoa has three main pillars: early detection of NCDs, NCD management, and increased community awareness. The model takes advantage of existing community structures where extended families continue to play a significant role in daily life and culture. Each village in Samoa has a women's committee representative whose role is to liaise with government agencies to facilitate early NCD detection.
>
> In communities where the pilot has been implemented, over 92% of the target population has now been reached, thanks in large part to efforts by women's committee representatives to inform and encourage villagers to participate. Of those screened, 12.7% of people aged over 40 years have been tested and found to have hyperglycaemia. Through the PEN Fa'a Samoa implementation, members of the community with abnormal results are referred to a management team at the district health facility and seen by a physician who discusses a management and treatment plan with them, and prescribes medication and behaviour changes. Trained community women representatives then help patients carry out their treatment plan. The Ministry of Health and the National Health Service, with the support of WHO, aim to replicate PEN Fa'a Samoa in more villages on the island to achieve full implementation by the end of 2016.

3.2 MANAGEMENT OF DIABETES — CORE COMPONENTS

People with diabetes require access to systematic, ongoing and organized care delivered by a team of skilled health-care providers. Outcomes can be improved at the primary care level with basic interventions involving medication, health education and counselling, and consistent follow-up. This systematic care should include a periodic review of metabolic control and complications, an agreed and continually updated diabetes care plan, and access to person-centred care provided by a multidisciplinary team. New technologies such as telemedicine and mobile phone technology are also increasingly being used and have the potential to reach remote areas (see Box 7).

While most treatment and tests can be done at primary care level, periodic referral for specialist care is required, for example, for comprehensive eye examinations, laser and surgical treatment of eye complications, complex kidney function tests, and tests of the heart and arteries in the limbs. All cases of acute cardiovascular disease, diabetic coma, kidney failure and infected foot ulcers should be managed in a hospital.

> **BOX 7. IMPROVING DIABETES MANAGEMENT USING MOBILE TECHNOLOGY**
>
> SMS-based programmes can contribute to the prevention and management of diabetes in a way that is acceptable to patients and the general population. Interventions studied span the disease spectrum, using one-way and two-way SMS messages to provide information, medication reminders, and increase patient-provider communication.
>
> Reviews of existing clinical studies indicate that text messaging can be effective in promoting positive health behaviour change and disease management for people with diabetes *(10)*. When properly designed, mobile diabetes support has generated a statistically significant improvement in areas such as patient glycaemic control in the short-term and long-term (over 6 months), and medication adherence *(11, 12)*.
>
> **The mRamadan initiative, Senegal**
>
> During Ramadan, a lack of understanding of safe ways to manage the fasting tradition can lead to severe health problems and complications for people with diabetes. Every year during Ramadan, health authorities in Senegal witness a peak in the urgent hospitalization of people with uncontrolled diabetes.
>
> The Government of Senegal was keen to use mobile technology to improve access to support during Ramadan for people with diabetes, and began a programme in 2014 with technical support from WHO and the International Telecommunications Union (ITU). The programme sent SMS tips and advice to enrolled diabetics during Ramadan to promote good health behaviours during and between fasting periods. This included reminders for people to drink at least 1 litre of water each morning before beginning the fast; information for health-care providers on medication use; and which foods to avoid when breaking a fast in the evening. In a qualitative review, users reported it as a helpful source of support. When the mRamadan programme was run in 2015 for a second round the programme saw 12 000 self-recruited users, highlighting demand and the potential for further expansion.

National guidelines and management protocols developed for (or adapted to) individual settings are useful tools in achieving a standardized and consistent management approach. They should cover these basic principles of diabetes management:

- Interventions to promote and support healthy lifestyles, including healthy diet, physical activity, avoidance of tobacco use and harmful use of alcohol.

- Medication for blood glucose control – insulin or oral hypoglycaemic agents as required.

- Medication to control cardiovascular disease risk.

- Regular exams for early detection of complications: comprehensive eye examination[1], measurement of urine protein, and assessment of feet for signs of neuropathy.

- Standard criteria for referral of patients from primary care to secondary or tertiary care.

---

1. Comprehensive eye examination includes visual acuity, intraocular pressure measurement and dilated examination of the retina and the optic nerve head, with retinal imaging strongly recommended.

- Integrated management of diabetes and other diseases (see Diabetes and other NCDs, page 55).

The effectiveness of diabetes management ultimately depends on people's compliance with recommendations and treatment. Patient education is therefore an important component of diabetes management. Patients need to understand the principles and importance of a healthy diet, adequate physical activity, avoidance of tobacco and harmful use of alcohol, adherence to medication, foot hygiene and appropriate footwear, and the need for periodic assessment of metabolic control and the presence or progression of complications *(13)*.

INTERVENTIONS TO PROMOTE HEALTHIER EATING AND PHYSICAL ACTIVITY

All people with diabetes need counselling on healthy diet and regular physical activity, adapted to their capabilities. Existing guidelines for dietary management of type 2 diabetes do not give identical recommendations, but all agree on: a lower calorie intake for overweight and obese patients, and replacing saturated fats with unsaturated fats *(14)*; intake of dietary fibre equal to or higher than that recommended for the general population *(15)*; and avoiding added sugars, tobacco use and excessive use of alcohol *(16)*. Education of patients in groups is a cost-effective strategy *(13)*.

It has been suspected for some time that energy restriction through a very low-calorie diet can lead to the reduction of symptoms or to the reversal of hyperglycaemia typical of type 2 diabetes – the reversal may be maintained so long as weight is not regained *(17)* (see Box 8).

Energy restriction through bariatric (or metabolic) surgery to reduce the size of the stomach is now established as an effective treatment for severe obesity-related type 2 diabetes, at least in communities and health-care contexts where necessary resources are available. The disappearance of diabetes that occurs in a large number of diabetic patients after bariatric surgery often happens within days of surgery, similar to that which occurs at the start of a very low-calorie diet, before weight loss – indicating the possible role of gut-related hormones in glucose metabolism. Depending on the surgical technique, reduction in excess body weight ranges from 54–72% *(18)*. However, many health-care settings lack the required resources for this type of surgery, making such treatment accessible to only a few.

In addition to general health benefits, physical activity appears to have a beneficial effect on insulin action, blood glucose control and metabolic abnormalities associated with diabetes. Physical activity can also be beneficial in reducing cardiovascular disease risk factors. Activity should be regular and ideally combine aerobic exercise with resistance training *(19)*.

> **Blood glucose control is important in preventing and slowing the progression of complications**

BOX 8. REVERSING TYPE 2 DIABETES, BARBADOS

Barbados has a 19% prevalence of diabetes among adults. One in three adults is obese; two out of three are overweight or obese; and under one in 10 adults eats five or more portions of fresh fruit and vegetables a day.

The Barbados Diabetes Reversal Study is designed to test the feasibility of an 8-week, low-calorie diet, with follow-up support for 6 months on diet and physical activity, to reverse type 2 diabetes.

Ten men and 15 women aged 26–68 years participated in the study. All had been diagnosed with type 2 diabetes in the previous 6 years, none was on insulin, and their body mass indices ranged from 27–53. All glucose-lowering medication ceased at the start of the study. Participants consumed a predominantly liquid diet consisting of four portions a day, each of 190 calories. Participants were also encouraged to eat low-carbohydrate, high-fibre vegetables.

By week 8, average weight loss was 10 kg. Several people saw improvements in blood glucose levels and in blood pressure. Three months after finishing the 8-week diet, 17 participants had fasting plasma glucose (FPG) below the diagnostic threshold for diabetes compared to three at the start, and despite remaining off glucose-lowering medication. For nine of the 12 participants on medication for hypertension at the start of the study, blood pressure fell sufficiently that they could stop taking hypertension medication by the 8th week.

Participants have so far articulated several challenges in participating in the study, including the monotony of the low-calorie diet phase, the high cost of fresh fruits and vegetables, and feeling poorly equipped to prepare non-starchy vegetables, even with provided recipes. There was resounding agreement that the most challenging times are in social settings, where there is peer pressure to consume food and drink.

A key element of the programme's success has been the support participants have received from family, friends and each other (particularly through the use of social media). However, their experiences also demonstrate the everyday difficulties of undertaking this approach in a context of widespread obesity.

BLOOD GLUCOSE CONTROL

The role of blood glucose control in preventing the development and progression of complications has been proven in both type 1 and type 2 diabetes, with an especially strong relationship between intensive blood glucose control and neuropathy and diabetic retinopathy *(20, 21)*. In most patients with diabetes, blood glucose levels can be adequately managed with medicines included in the *WHO Model list of essential medicines (22)*. These are metformin, gliclazide, and short-acting and intermediate-acting human or animal insulin.

Blood glucose control should be monitored through regular measurement. People with type 1 diabetes and gestational diabetes need strict control of blood glucose which is difficult to accomplish and monitor in primary health care, so they will need more frequent referral to higher levels of health care.

Glycated haemoglobin (HbA1c) is the method of choice for

monitoring glycaemic control in diabetes. An advantage of using HbA1c is that the patient does not need to be in a fasting state. Ideally it should be measured twice a year in people with type 2 diabetes and more frequently in those with type 1 diabetes. However, HbA1c testing is more costly than glucose measurement, and therefore less readily available. If HbA1c testing is not available, fasting or post-meal blood glucose is an acceptable substitute.

Self-monitoring of blood glucose is recommended for patients receiving insulin, and to have a plan of action with their health provider on how to adjust insulin dosage, food intake and physical activity according to their blood glucose levels. Availability of self-monitoring devices and strips has not been assessed globally. Anecdotal evidence suggests that self-monitoring is not available for a vast majority of people on insulin treatment – cost being cited as the most frequent reason. Some data indicate that less costly self-monitoring by urine glucose measurement could be an acceptable alternative when blood glucose self-monitoring is not possible (23).

MEDICATION FOR ASSOCIATED CARDIOVASCULAR DISEASE RISK FACTORS

Comprehensive reduction of cardiovascular disease risk factors, including the control of blood pressure and lipids in addition to blood glucose, is of vital importance in preventing the development of cardiovascular disease in diabetes, but also in preventing microvascular complications. This can be achieved with generic medicines from *WHO Model list of essential medicines* (22) (thiazide diuretic, ACE-inhibitor, beta blockers, statin).

SCREENING FOR EARLY DETECTION AND TREATMENT OF COMPLICATIONS

Current treatment of diabetes does not prevent all complications, but the progress of complications can be slowed by early interventions (13). People with diabetes should have periodic, comprehensive eye examinations. Timely laser photocoagulation and good control of blood glucose can prevent or delay the onset of irreversible vision loss, though this is not always accessible or available in low- and middle-income countries. Measurement of urine protein will reveal early kidney damage, and the progression to kidney failure can be slowed by essential drugs routinely used to treat hypertension. Kidney failure is treated by dialysis or a kidney transplant. Proper footwear and regular examination of feet for signs of neuropathy, impaired blood flow and skin changes can prevent foot ulcers that often lead to gangrene and limb amputation. Rehabilitation services such as physiotherapy and occupational therapy can help minimize the impact of complications on people's functioning (see Box 9).

HUMAN RESOURCES

A range of health professionals is required for the care and treatment of diabetes, including physicians, nurses, dieticians and specialists such as obstetricians, ophthalmologists, vascular surgeons and physiotherapists.

> **BOX 9. REHABILITATION FOLLOWING DIABETES-RELATED AMPUTATION, TAJIKISTAN**
>
> The physical complications associated with diabetes, including poor vascularization, can cause lower-limb wounds that may lead to amputation. Without proper care and support this can profoundly limit a person's ability to work, play a full family role and enjoy recreational activities. Furthermore, people with diabetic wounds require close attention to prevent infection and deterioration that can lead to death. Rehabilitation services play a fundamental role across the continuum of care for people with diabetes, helping prevent complications and providing interventions to keep people mobile and active.
>
> Approximately half of the 5000 people with diabetes that report to Tajikistan's Republican Endocrinology Hospital every year require rehabilitation services. The International Committee of the Red Cross/Special Fund for the Disabled provides technical support to Tajikistan's only physical rehabilitation centre, which provides multidisciplinary care to people with diabetes and associated complications.
>
> The team of physiotherapists, prosthetists and social workers, provide holistic interventions that help people work and participate in society. Key aspects of their interventions include:
>
> - assessment and provision of assistive devices;
> - physical rehabilitation, including strengthening, endurance and gait training for those with lower-limb amputations;
> - facilitating return to work;
> - providing education on self-management to prevent deterioration.
>
> While the rehabilitation service has seen encouraging outcomes (increasing functional independence, participation in society and continuation of livelihood) in the lives of people with diabetes, knowledge of rehabilitation services among the public and all levels of the health-care system remains poor. Work is being done to increase the awareness of rehabilitation services and the important role they play in diabetic care.

But in many settings, access to even the most basic health professionals with appropriate training in diabetes management is not available. While more and better-trained health professionals could rectify this problem, in many situations it is not a realistic solution. However there are examples of innovative solutions, including up-skilling available health professionals to deliver diabetes care (see Box 10) and training lay people to deliver protocol-driven care. WHO PEN includes management protocols for non-medically qualified health-care workers.

3.3 INTEGRATED MANAGEMENT OF DIABETES AND OTHER CHRONIC HEALTH CONDITIONS

Diabetes management should be integrated with management of other NCDs, and in some settings tuberculosis and HIV/AIDS, to improve equity, efficiency and outcomes. Diabetes is frequently comorbid with a range of other diseases and conditions, the interactions of which have an impact on its management. In addition to cardiovascular diseases, ageing-related conditions such as cognitive decline and physical disability have emerged as frequent comorbid conditions with diabetes. Depression is two to three times more common in people with diabetes than in those without, for example *(24)*.

The epidemiological transition occurring in many low- and middle-income countries is characterized by the coexistence of established infectious disease alongside emerging NCD epidemics *(25)*. Some of these diseases interact, mediated by shared risk factors *(25)*, and their management may be complicated by drug-disease and drug-drug interactions. The increasing longevity of people with HIV/AIDS, for example, is accompanied by a rising incidence and prevalence of insulin resistance and type 2 diabetes among them, some of which may be related to antiretroviral treatment *(25, 26)*.

DIABETES AND OTHER NCDs

Diabetes has close links with other NCDs and their risk factors. Recommended management of high cardiovascular disease risk, for

---

BOX 10. BUILDING CAPACITY FOR DIABETES MANAGEMENT, THAILAND

The increasing burden of diabetes and the demand for better care have made capacity-building essential for Thailand's recently introduced diabetes management system and practice guidelines. The system includes diabetes risk assessment and screening; assessment of chronic complications and their risks; and clinical care schemes in primary, secondary and tertiary care settings with a referral system and designated outcome indicators.

There are regular training courses for building capacity. Basic training courses (3 to 5 days) are implemented by the Diabetes Association of Thailand and the Thai Society of Diabetes Educators for diabetes care teams, including nurses, dietitians, pharmacists and physiotherapists. Over the past 10 years this course has trained more than 6000 health-care providers. A 4-month training course for nurses responsible for managing diabetes has been established by the Thailand Nursing and Midwifery Council and Faculty of nursing, Mahidol University. Currently, there are more than 1000 disease-manager nurses. In addition, a 5-day camp for practicing physicians treating type 1 diabetes is run by the Diabetes Association of Thailand and the Endocrine Society of Thailand, alongside annual scientific meetings.

Thailand's Ministry of Public Health has developed the "simple diabetes care" concept for village and district public health volunteers to enable them to visit patients at home and encourage their adherence to medical advice, treatment and regular follow-up appointments. This has lowered the rate of undiagnosed cases from 53% to 31%; increased the number of patients attending health-care facilities; and increased the annual rate of vascular risk assessments and detection of early stage of chronic diabetic complications. A specific training course for foot and wound care has resulted in a declining rate of foot ulcers and amputations. Capacity-building of care teams in providing standard care for diabetes in children and adolescents is now underway.

example, includes blood glucose control and counselling (for healthy diet and physical activity), and, similarly, management of diabetes includes anti-hypertensive medications at lower levels of blood pressure than for non-diabetics *(13)*. An organized and integrated health system is necessary to deliver optimal diabetes care. Relatively simple measures can be implemented, including standard protocols and clear referral pathways between different health-care providers and different levels of care.

A core set of such interventions is defined in the WHO PEN package, which includes interventions for detection, prevention, treatment and care of diabetes, cardiovascular disease, chronic respiratory disease and cancer through a primary health-care approach *(13)*. They are evidence-based, cost-effective and feasible for implementation – even in low-resource settings. WHO PEN equips both physicians and non-physician health workers in primary care.

WHO PEN specifies the minimum essential resources needed to implement its protocols: cardiovascular risk prediction charts, essential medicines and basic technologies, and costing tools for decision-makers. WHO PEN also guides policy-makers in the assessment of health system gaps and the process of the patient visit, including prescribing medication, the content of counselling and the frequency of follow-ups. Explicit criteria for referral to higher levels of care are provided. A simplified medical record stores key information in an organized way and serves as a reminder to follow-up actions that should be taken at each visit.

If effectively implemented, WHO PEN can strengthen health systems, improve the quality of NCD (including diabetes) care, and support the attainment of global NCD targets (see Box 1, page 16) WHO PEN implementation may facilitate post-disaster health system recovery and provide continuity of care for people with NCDs. The swift implementation of WHO PEN in the Philippines following Typhoon Haiyan in 2013 resulted in increased availability of trained health service providers; improved availability of essential equipment, supplies and medicines; functional referral systems; and the use of monitoring tools, within 3 months *(27)*.

DIABETES AND TUBERCULOSIS

Diabetes is a known risk factor for tuberculosis *(28)* and is associated with poorer tuberculosis outcomes, while tuberculosis is associated with worsening glycaemic control *(29)*. Since a number of countries have both a high and increasing diabetes prevalence and a substantial burden of tuberculosis, this interaction has significant implications for management of both diseases.

Active bi-directional screening has been reported to be associated with the detection of more tuberculosis and diabetes *(30)* and there have been reports of the successful piloting and implementation of bi-directional screening policies. For example, in India, a pilot study demonstrated the feasibility of screening tuberculosis patients for type 2 diabetes *(31)*, and the National Tuberculosis Programme was subsequently revised to implement this intervention across India.

WHO's Collaborative Framework for Care and Control of Tuberculosis and Diabetes provides guidelines to establish mechanisms of collaboration, including joint coordination, bi-directional surveillance and screening of tuberculosis and type 2 diabetes, and guidelines for detection and management of diabetes in tuberculosis patients (and vice versa) *(32)*.

REORIENTING HEALTH SYSTEMS

Many health-care systems have evolved to respond to acute, infectious disease and are not organized to manage the demographic and epidemiogic transition towards noncommunicable diseases. The presence of lifelong or long-term comorbidities requires not just a rethinking of service delivery but also a reorientation of the entire health system in order to rise to the challenge of joint management of diabetes and other diseases. Expanding universal health coverage and access to integrated, people-centred health services would facilitate this reorientation.

Universal health coverage aims to ensure that all people have access to health promotion, preventive, curative and rehabilitative health services of sufficient quality to be effective, while also ensuring that people do not suffer financial hardship when paying for these services. People should not be forced into poverty because of the cost of health care, like the catastrophic personal health expenditure required of many people with diabetes. Inclusion of diabetes-related services in universal health coverage provides patient protection.

All countries can take action to move more rapidly towards universal health coverage. Key factors in determining which services are prioritized by countries are the epidemiological context, health systems development, levels of socioeconomic development and people's expectations. There is considerable diversity in health-care systems around the world and systems need to be flexible, locally adaptable, innovative and accessible to address the increasing challenge of diabetes and other diseases.

Moving away from the compartmentalization of health services, or "silos," towards integrated health services is a way to improve care and also to advance universal health coverage by increasing the efficiency and effectiveness of service delivery. The total cardiovascular disease (CVD) risk approach, for example, enables integrated management of hypertension, diabetes and other cardiovascular risk factors in primary care, and targets available resources at those most likely to develop heart attacks, strokes and diabetes complications *(33)*. Integrated health services can deliver a continuum of health promotion, disease prevention, diagnosis, treatment, rehabilitation and palliative care services, through the different levels and sites of care within the health system over the course of a lifetime.

> **People should not be forced into poverty because of the cost of diabetes care**

Orienting these services around people's needs, not just diseases, and approaching them as participants of care, not just beneficiaries, will help ensure that people receive the right care at the right time. WHO's *Global strategy on people-centred and integrated health services* outlines different pathways to empower and engage people; to strengthen health governance and accountability; to reorient the model of health-care services; to coordinate services; and to create an enabling environment *(34)*.

3.4 ACCESS TO ESSENTIAL MEDICINES AND BASIC TECHNOLOGIES

All people with type 1 diabetes, and many with type 2, require medication to reduce their blood glucose levels. A discussion of diabetes management must therefore include a closer look at access to essential medicines and basic technologies.

An increasing number of costly blood-glucose lowering medications are becoming available, but WHO's *Model list of essential medicines* contains effective, established and cost-effective treatments that should form the basis of therapeutic options. This applies not just for low- and middle-income resource settings but high-income settings too, as there is the chance that expenditure on non-essential medicines in these countries may contribute to catastrophic health expenditure *(35, 36)*. Availability in public health-care settings can depend on the inclusion of the medicine on countries' National Essential Medicines Lists (NEML), and whether the NEML serves as basis for procurement, training of staff, reimbursement systems and prescription decisions.

Governments should secure funding for essential medicines and technologies to diagnose and manage diabetes. Affordability depends mainly on the use of generic medicines and their use should be promoted – and their quality assured – through a strong national regulatory system. Responsible use of medicines can be promoted by the implementation of evidence-based guidelines and treatment protocols. Along with better procurement and policies for generic substitution, affordability for patients or for the system (if medicines are given free to patients or if a national health insurance system is in place) could be improved by regulation of mark-ups in the supply chain, and tax or tariff exemption (see Box 11).

INSULIN AND ORAL HYPOGLYCAEMIC AGENTS

People with type 1 diabetes require insulin for survival – without insulin, even for a short time, these individuals may face life-threatening consequences. Yet an array of international and national barriers interact to hamper access to insulin, and many in low- and middle-income countries do not receive this essential treatment *(39, 40)*.

The insulin market is dominated by a small number of multinational manufacturers, with a few, smaller producers making up only 4% of the market by volume *(41)*. This limited competition can potentially

> **BOX 11. IMPROVING ACCESS TO INSULIN AND ORAL MEDICINES FOR DIABETES, MOLDOVA**
>
> Although insulin is on WHO's *Model list of essential medicines*, access in resource-poor settings can still be a problem because of international and national barriers – not just because of costs but also because of access issues.
>
> The Republic of Moldova – where around one in eight adults (12.3% of the population) has diabetes or reduced tolerance to glucose *(37)* – has tried to address these issues within its broader health systems strengthening. Financial access to services improved with the introduction of mandatory health insurance in 2002, which became fully operational in 2004. Health expenditure as a percentage of state budget has increased to an appropriate and stable level. There has been an expansion of coverage of basic health services, enabling universal access to primary health care and pre-hospital emergency care, and additional benefits introduced to expand coverage to drugs prescribed in outpatient settings.
>
> Positive developments in the last decade relating to pharmaceuticals that are of relevance to diabetes include: increased funding for public reimbursement of outpatient drugs; introduction of external reference pricing; inclusion of insulin in the list of reimbursed drugs since 2013; and introduction of mandatory generic prescribing *(38)*. All Moldovan citizens are now entitled to free access to oral medicines for diabetes and insulin: there are three types of insulin and four oral medicines for diabetes that are 100% reimbursable.
>
> Previously, insulin shortages had been reported by both patient representatives and doctors which were thought to be the result of distribution problems, ineffective systems for monitoring stock levels, and the high number of tests required by the quality control system that caused delays in supply. There has been a change in the procurement of insulin since 2013, with a move from a national tender programme to decentralized procurement by pharmacies. In principle, such a move was expected to lead to several positive changes: a more reliable supply; increased choice of insulin types; greater availability across the country; and shorter travel times for patients.
>
> There is still some way to go but the general view of clinicians and patients is that great progress has been made. The Republic of Moldova has also recognised that access to medicines needs to be addressed in parallel to creating a health system able to manage all aspects of diabetes care.

increase insulin prices. Additional factors in the insulin market that may impact price include different insulin formulations coming off-patent, as well as the considerable increase in use of analogue insulin. Both of these factors affect the price of insulin before it ever arrives in a given country. Figure 6 shows that low-income countries generally pay most for insulin while high and middle-income countries pay least *(42)*.

Governments' decisions about insulin purchasing– tendering practices, choice of supplier, choice of products and delivery devices – can have a huge impact on budgets and on costs to end users. Governments may recoup high costs by charging mark-ups to patients. In Mozambique, for example, insulin purchased from local wholesalers was 25% to 125% more expensive than that purchased through international tenders *(43)*. In

FIGURE 6. MEDIAN ANNUAL PRICES FOR A 10 ML VIAL OF 100 IU INSULIN DURING 2003–2014, BY COUNTRY INCOME GROUP

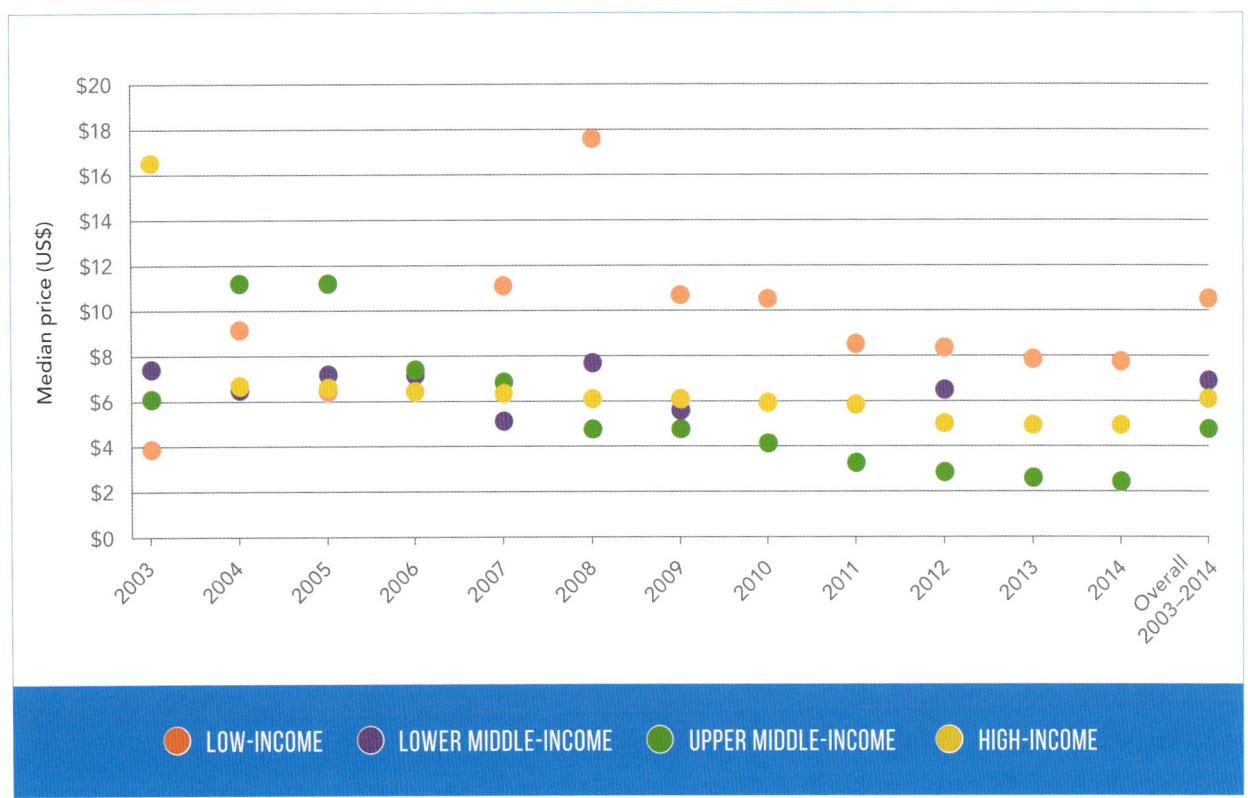

Source: International Drug Price Indicator Guide (see Annex B for methods).

Kyrgyzstan, purchasing insulin in cartridges (analogue insulin), cost the ministry of health 2.5 to 8.5 times the costs that would have accrued if the purchase had aligned with WHO's *Model list of essential medicines (44)*.

Mark-ups throughout the system, ranging from import tariffs, value added taxes, pharmacy costs and storage and transportation costs further increase the cost to individuals. An assessment of insulin affordability found that 1 month of insulin treatment would cost the lowest-paid government worker the equivalent of 2.8 days of work in Brazil, 4.7 days in Pakistan, 6.1 days in Sri Lanka, 7.3 days in Nepal, and 19.6 days in Malawi *(45)*. Distribution factors also affect availability. For example, insulin supplies may remain in the capital city or major urban areas when proper cold chain management makes transfer of supplies to other parts of the country too expensive or cumbersome.

Other essential medicines for diabetes control – to improve blood glucose levels, blood pressure and lipid control – are frequently unavailable or intermittent, despite existence in generic form. In a study conducted in 40 low- and middle-income countries, glibenclamide and metformin were available in only 65% of private and 49.5% of public health-care facilities, and countries paid a median of 2.2 times more than the drug's international reference price *(46)*.

INJECTION DEVICES

Insulin must be injected, meaning syringes are also a survival need for people using insulin. Value added taxes are frequently applied to syringes, which are not readily available in the public sector. If syringes are purchased by the public sector, quantities are often insufficient and not linked to insulin purchases (6). Pen injection devices and insulin cartridges have some advantages over traditional syringes (being more practical when multiple daily injections of insulin are required) but their cost prohibits their use for many patients.

3.5 SUMMARY

A cluster of cost-effective interventions lies at the heart of improving diabetes outcomes: blood glucose control through a combination of diet, physical activity and, if necessary, medication; control of blood pressure and lipids to reduce cardiovascular risk and other complications; and regular screening and early intervention for damage to the eyes, kidneys and feet. This set of interventions appears simple but carrying them out depends on appropriate structures for health-care delivery such as access to essential medicines and technologies, protocols for management in primary care, appropriate training of health-care providers, referral systems involving specialists, and the active participation and motivation of the patient.

Currently, primary health-care services in many countries do not have the capacity to diagnose and manage diabetes (see Part 4). Building this capacity is a priority to achieve better outcomes for people with diabetes, and to meet global targets to halt the rise in obesity and diabetes and reduce premature mortality from NCDs. Diabetes management can be strengthened even in low-resource settings through implementation of the standards and protocols such as the WHO PEN package. Efforts to improve capacity for diagnosis and treatment of diabetes should be undertaken in the context of integrated NCD management. At a minimum, diabetes and cardiovascular disease management can be integrated. Integrated management of diabetes and TB and/or HIV/AIDS can be considered where there is high prevalence of these diseases.

Improving access to essential medicines is a vital aspect of achieving universal health coverage and of improving health systems' capacity to prevent and manage diabetes and other NCDs (47). Diabetes has been described as a tracer condition for assessing health system performance (48, 49) for many reasons: it is well-defined, fairly easy to diagnose, and common; and because optimal management of diabetes requires the coordinated involvement of a variety of health-care providers at multiple levels of the health-care system, ongoing monitoring, access to essential medicines and technologies, and active patient participation. Solutions for improving diabetes management could therefore provide lessons for management of other NCDs.

The costs of diabetes management are high but they are likely to be dwarfed by the economic costs of poor or non-existent care in the

> **Diabetes management can be strengthened through implementation of standards and protocols, even in low-resource settings**

future. National-level scaling-up of interventions that are either cost-saving or cost-effective would curb the increase of the future economic burden of the disease as well as significantly improve the quality of life for people with diabetes.

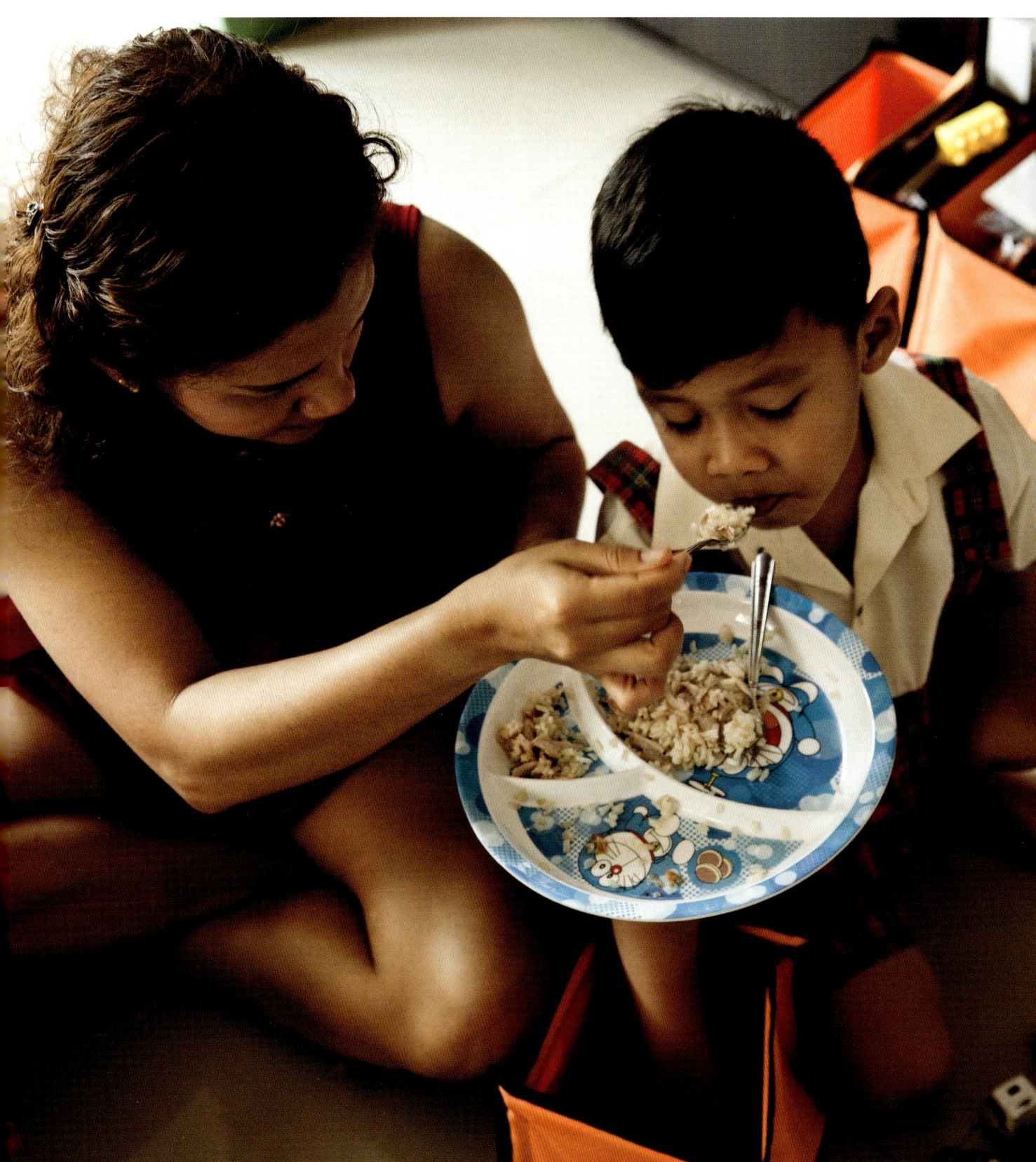

REFERENCES

1. Venkat Narayan KM, Zhang P, Kanaya AM, Williams DE, Engelgau MM, Imperatore G, et al. Diabetes: the pandemic and potential solutions. In: Disease control priorities in developing countries, 2 ed. Washington DC: World Bank; 2006:591–603.

2. Li R, Zhang P, Barker LE, Chowdhury FM, Zhang X. Cost-effectiveness of interventions to prevent and control diabetes mellitus: a systematic review. Diabetes Care. 2010;33:(8)1872–1894.

3. Williams DRR. The economics of diabetes care: a global perspective. In: International textbook of diabetes mellitus, 4th ed. Chichester, UK: Wiley Blackwell; 2015.

4. Harding JL, Shaw JE, Peeters A, Guiver T, Davidson S, Magliano DJ. Mortality trends among people with type 1 and type 2 diabetes in Australia: 1997–2010. Diabetes Care. 2014;37:(9)2579–2586.

5. Use of glycated haemoglobin (HbA1c) in the diagnosis of diabetes mellitus. Geneva: World Health Organization; 2011.

6. Beran D, Yudkin JS. Looking beyond the issue of access to insulin: what is needed for proper diabetes care in resource-poor settings. Diabetes Research and Clinical Practice. 2010;88:(3)217–221.

7. Herman WH, Ye W, Griffin SJ, Simmons RK, Davies MJ, Khunti K et al. Early detection and treatment of type 2 diabetes reduce cardiovascular morbidity and mortality: A simulation of the results of the Anglo-Danish-Dutch study of intensive treatment in people with screen-detected diabetes in primary care (ADDITION-Europe). Diabetes Care. 2015;38:(8)1449–1455.

8. Basu S, Millett C, Vijan S, Hayward RA, Kinra S, Ahuja R, et al. The health system and population health implications of large-scale diabetes screening in India: a microsimulation model of alternative approaches. PLoS.Med. 2015;12:(5) e1001827.

9. Screening for Type 2 diabetes. Report of a WHO and International Diabetes Federation meeting WHO/NMH/MNC/03.1. Geneva: World Health Organization; 2003.

10. Free C, Phillips G, Galli L, Watson L, Felix L, Edwards P, et al. The effectiveness of mobile-health technology-based health behaviour change or disease management interventions for health care consumers: a systematic review. PLoS Med. 2013;10:e1001362.

11. Liang X, Wang Q, Yang X, Cao J, Chen J, Mo X, et al. Effect of mobile phone intervention for diabetes on glycaemic control: a meta-analysis. Diabetes Medicine. 2011;28:455-463.

12. Vervloet, M., Dijk, L. van, Bakker, D.H. de, Souverein, P.C., Santen-Reestman, J., Vlijmen, B. van, Aarle, M.C.W. van, Hoek, L.S. van der, Bouvy, M.L. Short- and long-term effects of real-time medication monitoring with short message service (SMS) reminders for missed doses on the refill adherence of people with Type 2 diabetes: evidence from a randomised controlled trial. Diabetic Medicine: 2014, 31(7), 821-828.

13. Implementation tools: Package of Essential Noncommunicable (PEN) Disease Interventions for Primary Health Care in Low-Resource Settings. Geneva: World Health Organization; 2013.

14. Fats and fatty acids in human nutrition: report of an expert consultation. FAO Food and Nutrition Paper 91. Rome: Food and Agriculture Organization of the United Nations; 2010.

15. Ley SH, Hamdy O, Mohan V, Hu FB. Prevention and management of type 2 diabetes: dietary components and nutritional strategies. Lancet. 2014;383:(9933)1999–2007.

16. Guideline: Sugars intake for adults and children. Geneva: World Health Organization; 2015.

17. Taylor R. Type 2 diabetes: etiology and reversibility. Diabetes Care. 2013;36:(4)1047–1055.

18. Maggard-Gibbons M, Maglione M, Livhits M, Ewing B, Maher AR, Hu J, et al. Bariatric surgery for weight loss and glycemic control in non-morbidly obese adults with diabetes: a systematic review. Journal of the American Medical Association. 2013;309:(21)2250–2261.

19. Hayes C, Kriska A. Role of physical activity in diabetes management and prevention. Journal of the American Dietetic Association. 2008;108:(4 Suppl 1)S19–S23.

20. The effect of intensive treatment of diabetes on the development and progression of long-term complications in insulin-dependent diabetes mellitus. The Diabetes Control and Complications Trial Research Group. New England Journal of Medicine. 1993;329:(14)977–986.

21. Intensive blood-glucose control with sulphonylureas or insulin compared with conventional treatment and risk of complications in patients with type 2 diabetes (UKPDS 33). UK Prospective Diabetes Study (UKPDS) Group. Lancet. 1998;352:(9131)837–853.

22. WHO Model list of Essential Medicines. Geneva: World Health Organization; 2015.

23. Worth R, Home PD, Johnston DG, Anderson J, Ashworth L, Burrin JM, et al. Intensive attention improves glycaemic control in insulin-dependent diabetes without further advantage from home blood glucose monitoring: results of a controlled trial. British Medical Journal (Clinical Research Edition). 1982;285:(6350)1233–1240.

24. Roy T, Lloyd CE. Epidemiology of depression and diabetes: a systematic review. Journal of Affective Disorders. 2012;142:Suppl, S8-21.

25. Oni T, Youngblood E, Boulle A, McGrath N, Wilkinson RJ, Levit NS. Patterns of HIV, TB, and non-communicable disease multi-morbidity in peri-urban South Africa – a cross sectional study. BMC Infectious Diseases. 2015;15:20. doi:10.1186/s12879-015-0750-1.

26. Reid MJA, Tsima BM, Kirk B. HIV and diabetes in Africa. African Journal of Diabetes Medicine. 2012;20(2);28-32.

27. Martinez RE, Quintana R, Go JJ, Villones MS, Marquez MA. Use of the WHO Package of Essential Noncommunicable Disease Interventions after Typhoon Haiyan. Western Pacific Surveillance Response Journal. 2015;6:Suppl 1, 18–20.

28. Jeon CY, Murray MB. Diabetes mellitus increases the risk of active tuberculosis: a systematic review of 13 observational studies. PLoS Medicine. 2008;5:(7)e152.

29. Riza AL, Pearson F, Ugarte-Gil C, Alisjahbana B, van de Vijver S, Panduru NM, et al. Clinical management of concurrent diabetes and tuberculosis and the implications for patient services. Lancet Diabetes Endocrinology. 2014;2:(9)740–753.

30. Jeon CY, Harries AD, Baker MA, Hart JE, Kapur A, Lonnroth K, et al. Bi-directional screening for tuberculosis and diabetes: a systematic review. Tropical Medicine and International Health. 2010;15:(11)1300–1314.

31. Screening of patients with tuberculosis for diabetes mellitus in India. Tropical Medicine and International Health. 18;(5):636–645.

32. Collaborative framework for care and control of tuberculosis and diabetes. Geneva: World Health Organization; 2011.

33. Global status report on noncommunicable diseases. Geneva: World Health Organization; 2014.

34. WHO global strategy on people-centred and integrated health services. Interim report. Geneva: World Health Organization; 2015.

35. Luo J, Avorn J, Kesselheim AS. Trends in Medicaid reimbursements for insulin from 1991 through 2014. Journal of the American Medical Association Internal Medicine. 2015;175:(10)1681–1686.

36. Tylee T, Hirsch IB. Costs associated with using different insulin preparations. Journal of the American Medical Association. 2015;314:(7)665–666.

37. Republic of Moldova STEPS survey 2013: Fact sheet. Geneva: World Health Organization; 2014.

38. WHO Regional Office for Europe, Better noncommunicable disease outcomes: challenges and opportunities for health systems. Republic of Moldova country assessment. Copenhagen: World Health Organization; 2014.

39. Beran D. Improving access to insulin: what can be done? Diabetes Management. 2011;1:67–76.

40. Beran D, Perrin C, Billo N, Yudkin JS. Improving global access to medicines for non-communicable diseases. Lancet Global Health. 2014;2:(10)e561-e562.

41. Schultz K. The global diabetes care market. Novo Nordisk. 2011. Novo Nordisk.

42. International Drug Price Indicator Guide. Management Sciences for Health. Washington DC; Management Sciences for Health; 2015.

43. Beran D, Yudkin, JS, de Courten M. Access to care for patients with insulin-requiring diabetes in developing countries: case studies of Mozambique and Zambia. Diabetes Care. 2005;28:(9)2136–2140.

44. Beran D, Abdraimova A, Akkazieva B, McKee M, Balabanova D, Yudkin JS. Diabetes in Kyrgyzstan: changes between 2002 and 2009. International Journal of Health Planning Management. 2013;28:(2) e121-e137.

45. Mendis S, Fukino K, Cameron A, Laing R, Filipe A Jr, Khatib O, et al. The availability and affordability of selected essential medicines for chronic diseases in six low- and middle-income countries. Bulletin of the World Health Organization. 2007;85:(4)279–288.

46. Cameron A, Ewen M, Ross-Degnan D, Ball D, Laing R. Medicine prices, availability, and affordability in 36 developing and middle-income countries: a secondary analysis. Lancet. 2009;373:(9659)240–249.

47. Global action plan for the prevention and control of noncommunicable diseases 2013-2020. Geneva: World Health Organization; 2013.

48. Beran D, Yudkin J, de Courten M. Assessing health systems for type 1 diabetes in sub-Saharan Africa: developing a 'Rapid Assessment Protocol for Insulin Access.' BMC Health Services Research. 2006;6:17.

49. Nolte E, Bain C, McKee M. Diabetes as a tracer condition in international benchmarking of health systems. Diabetes Care. 2006;29(5):1007–11.

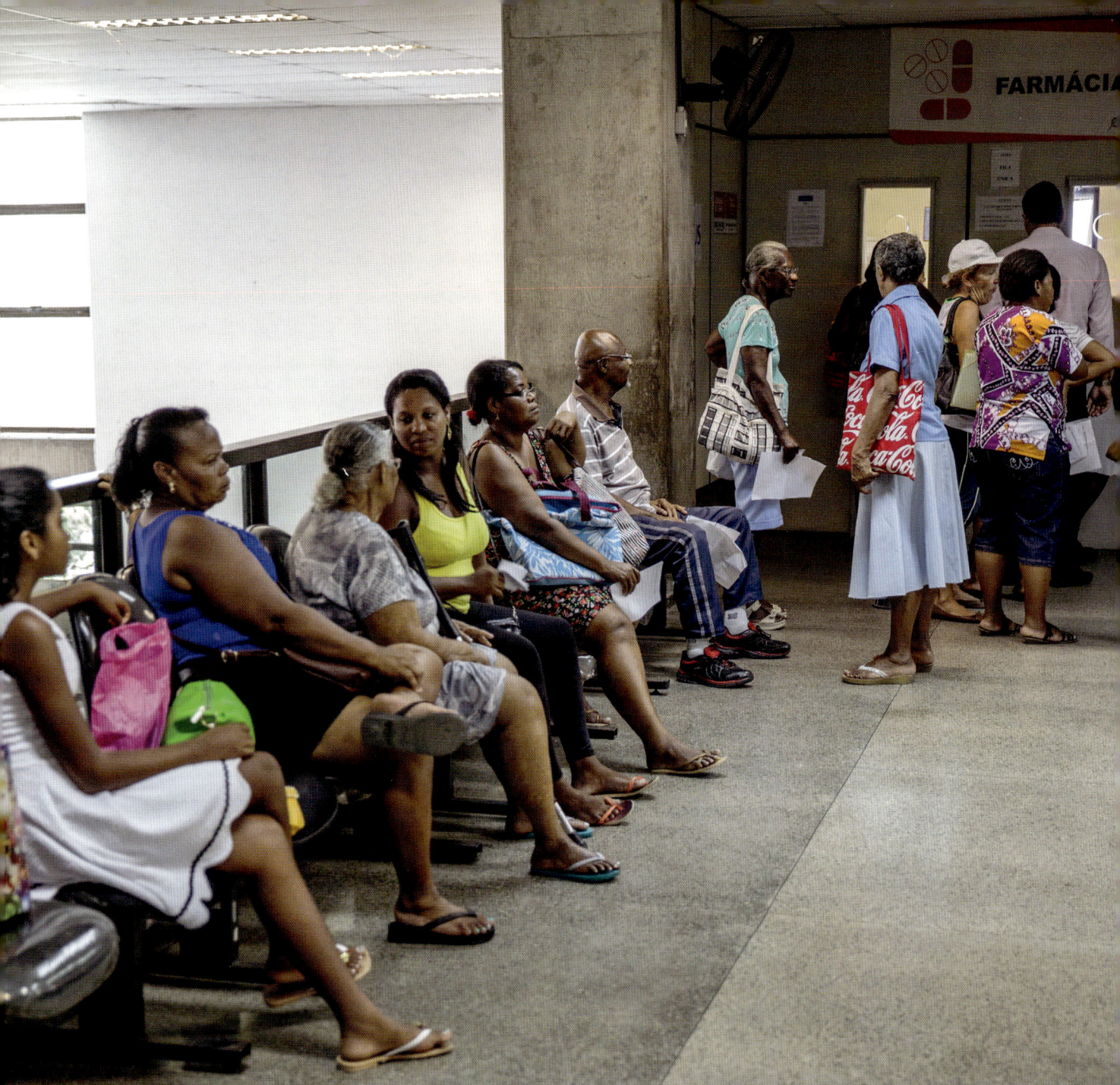

PART 4

NATIONAL CAPACITY FOR PREVENTION AND CONTROL OF DIABETES: A SNAPSHOT

KEY MESSAGES

The majority of countries have national diabetes policies, national policies to address unhealthy diet and physical inactivity, and national guidelines or standards for diabetes management.

Implementation and funding of national policies and guidelines is uneven.

Basic technologies for early detection, diagnosis and monitoring of diabetes in primary care settings are generally not available in low-income and lower middle-income countries.

Availability of insulin, metformin and sulphonylurea(s) is very limited in primary care facilities in low-income countries.

Less than half of countries have conducted a national, population-based survey with measurement of blood glucose status within the past 5 years.

This chapter provides a global snapshot of national capacity based on policies, plans and strategies for diabetes and its key risk factors; health system infrastructure such as guidelines for diabetes management in primary health care, availability of essential technologies for diagnosis and management, availability of essential medicines, and referral systems and treatment for complications; and surveillance. Such policies, plans and strategies contribute to the 10 progress indicators that will be used to report on progress towards implementation of national commitments outlined in the 2011 United Nations Political Declaration and the 2014 United Nations General Assembly Outcome Document on Noncommunicable Diseases *(1)*.

Data presented in this chapter come from the 2015 Noncommunicable Disease Country Capacity Survey (NCD CCS), to which national teams from 177 WHO Member States, representing 97% of the world's population, responded. The NCD CCS has been conducted regularly since 2000 to assess NCD governance and infrastructure, policy response, surveillance and health systems response at country level. It is increasingly used to monitor progress in achieving voluntary NCD targets and for reporting on NCD progress indicators *(2)*. There are limitations to the survey —for example its use of key informants rather than independently verified data collection — but on the whole it presents a clear picture of capacity and identifies areas that need more attention. Details of the survey methodology can be found in Annex B. Specific variables related to the prevention and management of diabetes are presented in this chapter. Individual profiles summarizing this data country by country are available online at *www.who.int/diabetes/global-report*.

4.1 NATIONAL POLICIES AND PLANS FOR DIABETES

Diabetes should be included in all national NCD policies to facilitate a coordinated, multisectoral response. Some countries might have a standalone policy or plan, some might include it in an integrated NCD policy, while others might do both.

Eighty-eight per cent of countries (156 countries) report having a national diabetes policy, plan or strategy. When funding and implementation are considered, however, a slightly different picture emerges. Seventy-two per cent of countries (127 countries) report having a national policy, plan, strategy or action plan on diabetes that is operational – i.e. one that has dedicated funding and is being implemented. In some regions and among some country-income levels, the proportion of countries whose policies, plans or strategies are operational shrinks (see Figure 7). Of the countries with operational national policies for diabetes, 44% (56 countries) include diabetes in an integrated NCD policy; 17% (22 countries) have a standalone policy for diabetes; and 39% (49 countries) do both.

FIGURE 7. PROPORTION OF COUNTRIES REPORTING OPERATIONAL AND NON-OPERATIONAL NATIONAL DIABETES POLICIES, BY WHO REGION AND COUNTRY INCOME GROUP

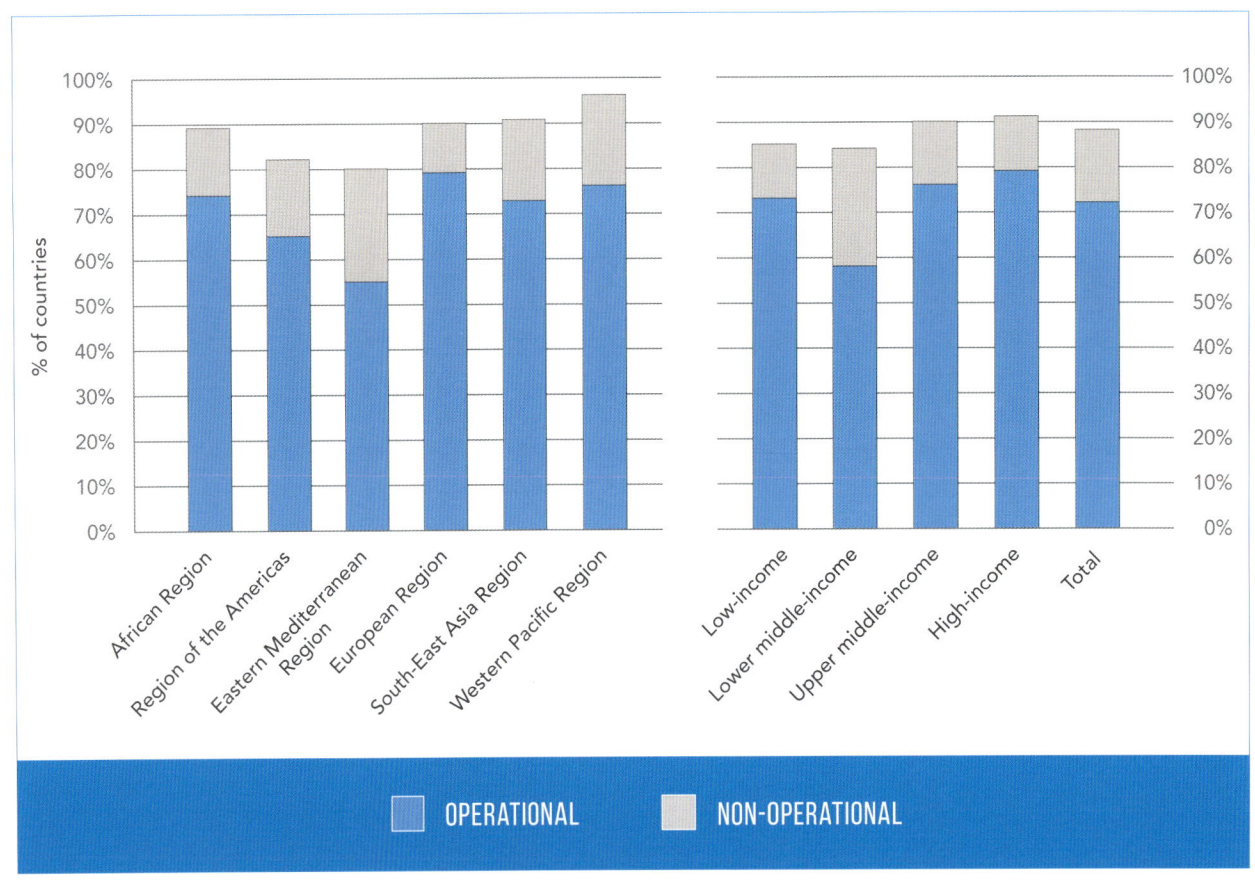

POLICIES RELATED TO PREVENTION

Key modifiable risk factors for the prevention of type 2 diabetes are overweight, obesity, physical inactivity and unhealthy diet (see Background section and Part 2). Most countries (89%) report having national policies addressing both healthy diet and physical activity, but when funding and implementation are considered, once again, the picture changes. About two thirds of countries (68%) report having operational policies addressing both healthy diet and physical activity, though this proportion varies by region and country income. Thirty-one per cent of countries report having operational policies to address overweight and obesity. High-income countries were more likely to report having operational policies in all of these areas than low- or middle-income countries, but it is worth noting that (encouragingly) the majority of low-income countries have operational policies to address diet and physical activity (see Figure 8).

4.2 NATIONAL GUIDELINES AND PROTOCOLS

National, evidence-based guidelines, protocols and standards for the management of diabetes are important tools for improving care. Overall, 71% of countries

68% of countries report having operational policies to address healthy diet and physical activity

FIGURE 8. PERCENTAGE OF COUNTRIES REPORTING OPERATIONAL POLICIES FOR SELECTED RISK FACTORS, BY WHO REGION AND COUNTRY INCOME GROUP

Note: policies include those that aim to reduce unhealthy diet and/or promote healthy diet, and those that aim to reduce physical inactivity and/or promote physical activity.

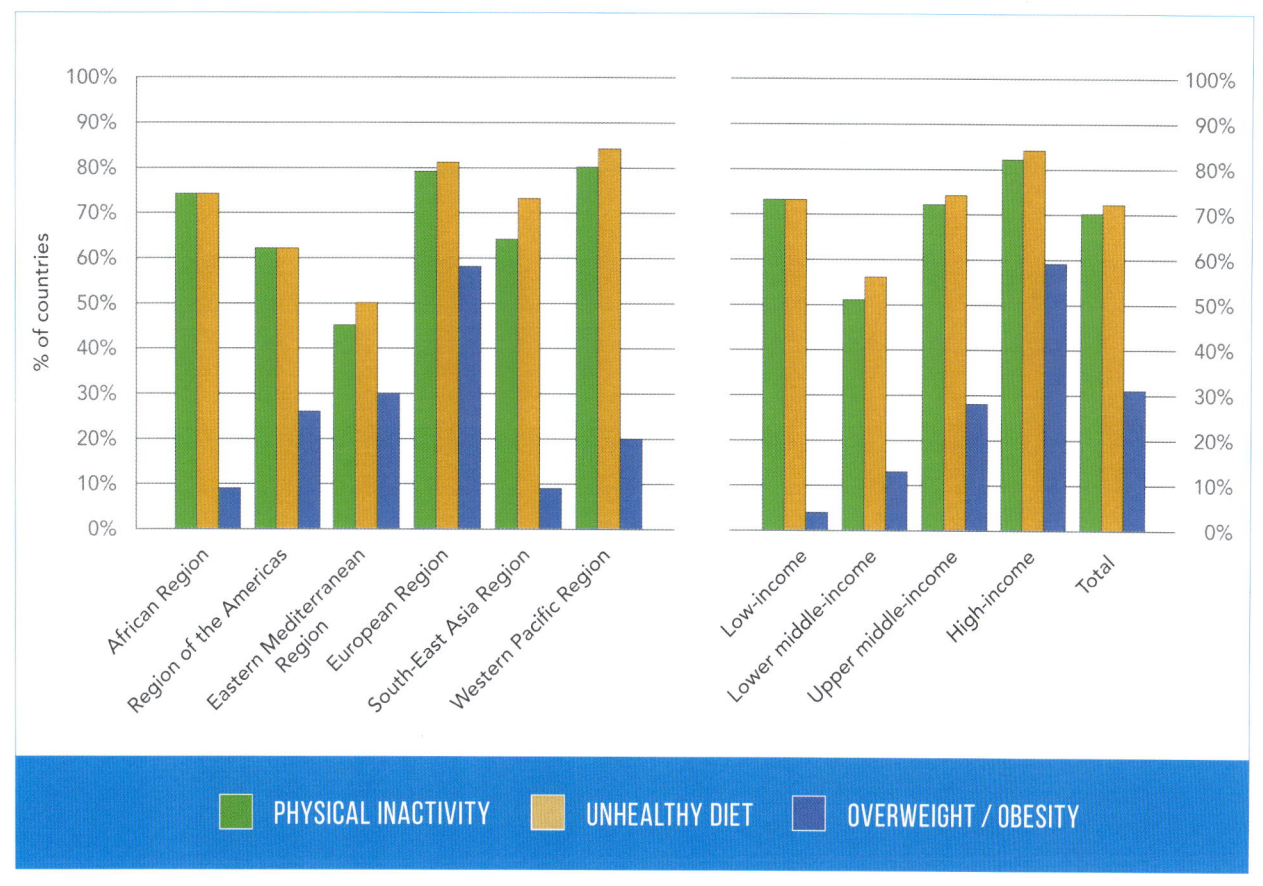

NATIONAL CAPACITY FOR PREVENTION AND CONTROL OF DIABETES: A SNAPSHOT   69

126 countries report having a national guideline for diabetes management that is partially or fully implemented

(126 countries) report having a national guideline for diabetes management that is either fully or partially implemented. Less than half of countries (47%) report full implementation. Middle- and high-income countries were more likely to report implementing guidelines for managing diabetes, with more than 70% reporting full or partial implementation (see Figure 9). Less than half (46%) of low-income countries reported fully or partially implementing diabetes management guidelines.

Diabetes management happens at different levels of the health-care delivery system. A referral system based on standard criteria contributes to continuity of care and ensures the optimal use of health-care services at different levels. Standard criteria for referral of patients from primary care to secondary or tertiary care were reported as available in 71% of countries (126 countries), but full implementation of such criteria was reported in only 42% of countries (74 countries). Full implementation of referral criteria is reported as achieved more often in upper middle-income and high-income countries, but even in these categories full implementation is not common (54% and 46% respectively).

FIGURE 9. PERCENTAGE OF COUNTRIES REPORTING FULLY OR PARTIALLY IMPLEMENTED DIABETES GUIDELINES, BY WHO REGION AND COUNTRY INCOME GROUP

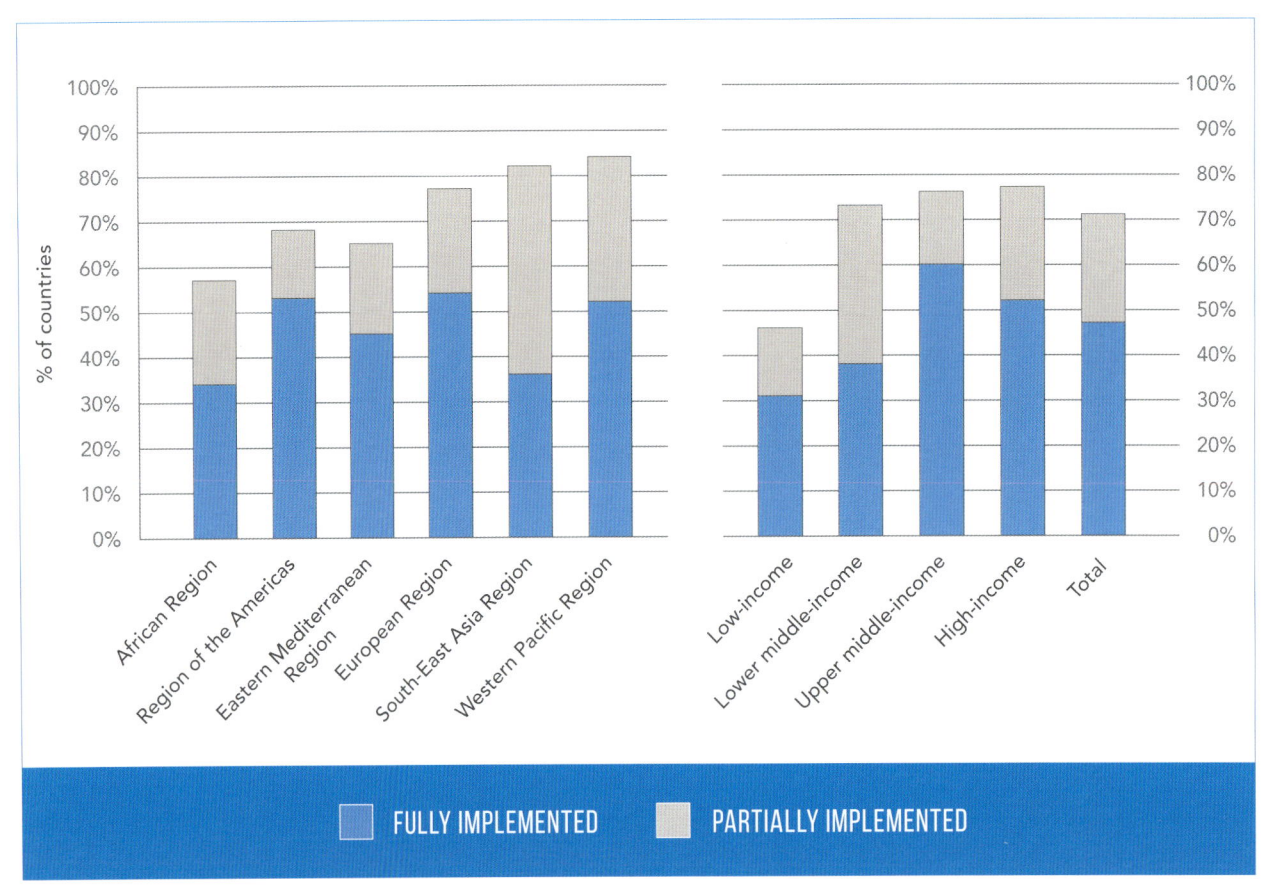

4.3 AVAILABILITY OF ESSENTIAL MEDICINES AND TECHNOLOGIES

The availability of essential medicines and basic technologies for early detection, diagnosis and monitoring of diabetes in primary health-care facilities is a critical component of management capacity. The NCD CCS asks the national team to rate the availability of essential medicines and basic technologies in primary care facilities. Items in question are rated "generally available" if they are available in 50% or more of primary care facilities in the country (or pharmacies, for medicines), otherwise they are rated "generally not available". The data in this section refer exclusively to availability within the publicly funded health-care sector and provide no indication of what may be available in the private health-care sector.

ESSENTIAL MEDICINES IN PRIMARY CARE FACILITIES

The NCD CCS includes availability of three essential medicines for diabetes management: insulin, metformin and sulphonylurea(s) (see Figure 10). Insulin was reported as generally available in 72% of countries (128 countries), but reported availability appears to vary widely by region and country income. Only 23% of low-income countries (six countries) report that insulin is generally available, in contrast to 96% of high-income

Only 23% of low-income countries report that insulin is generally available

FIGURE 10. PERCENTAGE OF COUNTRIES REPORTING ESSENTIAL MEDICINES ARE GENERALLY AVAILABLE IN PUBLICLY FUNDED PHARMACIES IN PRIMARY HEALTH-CARE FACILITIES

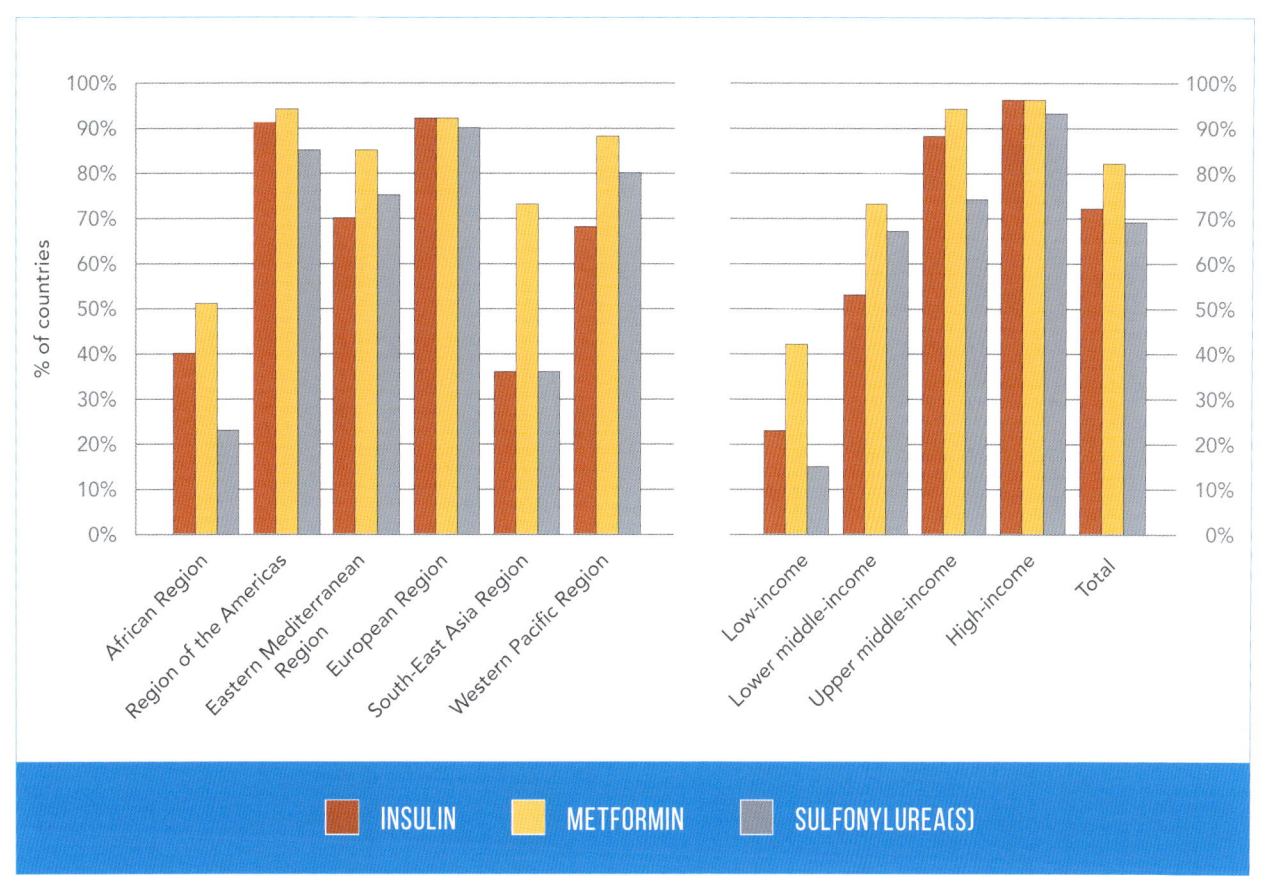

countries (54 countries). Further, the reported general availability of insulin in the WHO Region of the Americas and the European Region is more than double that of the WHO African Region and South-East Asia Region.

Regarding oral medications for glucose control, in 82% of countries (145 countries) metformin is reported as generally available, compared to 69% (123 countries) reporting general availability of sulphonylurea(s). Very few low-income countries report availability of both. Among high-income countries, more than 90% report that metformin and sulphonylurea(s) are generally available.

BASIC TECHNOLOGIES IN PRIMARY CARE FACILITIES

Essential technologies necessary for early detection, diagnosis and monitoring of diabetes in primary health care include weighing machines, measurement tapes, glucometers, blood glucose test strips, urine protein test strips and urine ketone test strips *(3)*.

Overall, 85% of countries (151 countries) report that blood glucose measurement is generally available in primary care settings, though this is true for only 50% of low-income countries (13 countries). Figure 11 shows the proportion of countries reporting general availability of height and weight measurement, blood glucose

> **Blood glucose measurement is reported as generally available in 50% of low-income countries**

FIGURE 11. PERCENTAGE OF COUNTRIES REPORTING BASIC TECHNOLOGIES GENERALLY AVAILABLE IN PUBLICLY-FUNDED PRIMARY HEALTH-CARE FACILITIES

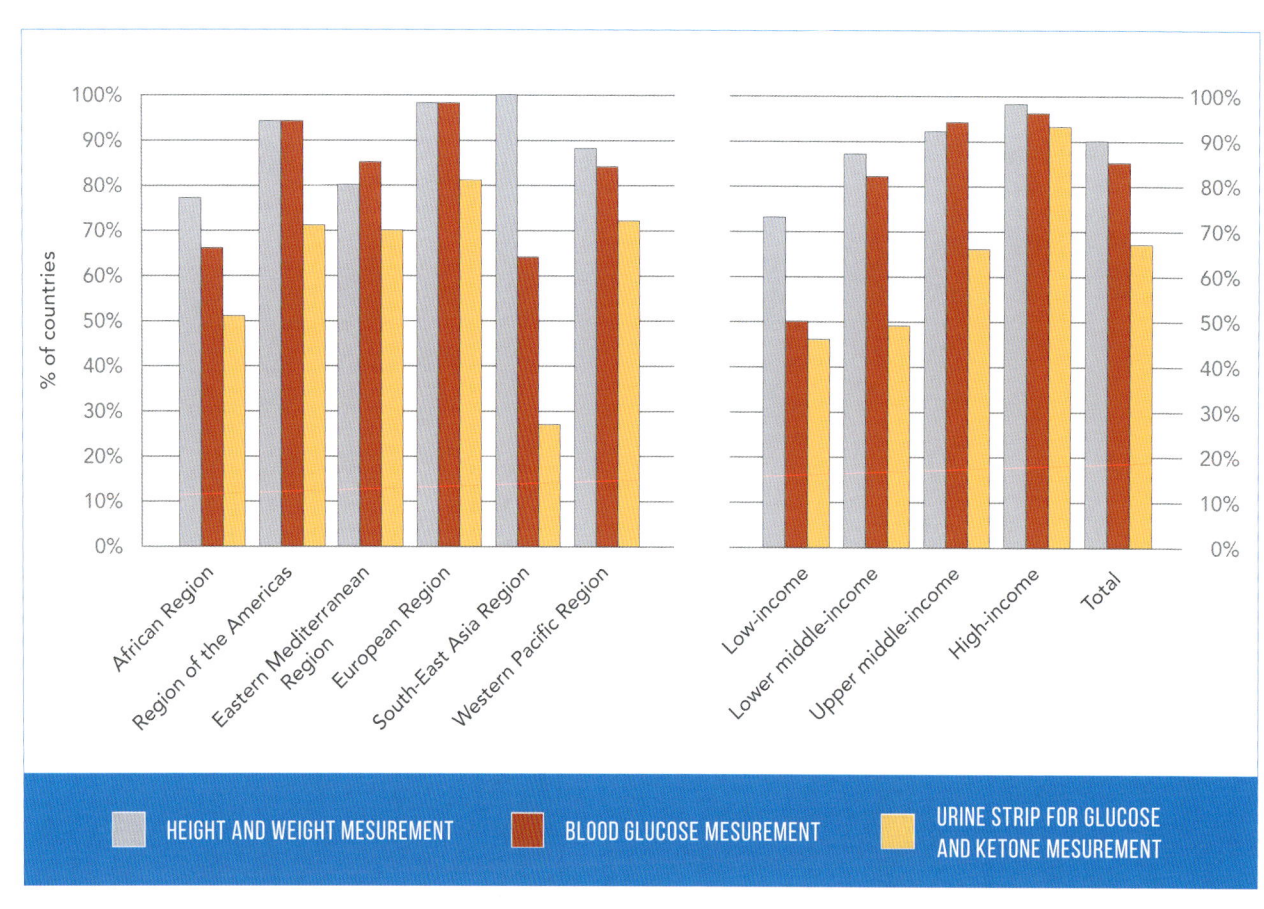

measurement, and urine strips for glucose and ketone measurement. There is a strong income gradient in reported availability of these essential technologies. Only one in three low-income and lower middle-income countries report having all three of these basic, essential technologies generally available, in contrast with nearly two in three of upper-middle and nearly all of high-income countries (not shown).

Figure 12 shows the reported availability of other, more expensive or sophisticated technologies and procedures useful for early detection, diagnosis and management of diabetes and its complications: oral glucose tolerance test, glycated haemoglobin (HbA1c) test, foot vibration by tuning fork, Doppler ultrasound testing of foot vascular status, and examination of the eye with dilated pupil (dilated fundus examination). It is clear that these additional technologies are much more readily available in high-income countries than in low- or middle-income countries.

MANAGEMENT OF KIDNEY FAILURE

Diabetes is a prominent cause of kidney disease. Kidney failure, also called end-stage renal disease, requires renal replacement therapy. Overall, 60% of countries (106 countries) reported general availability of renal replacement

FIGURE 12. PERCENTAGE COUNTRIES REPORTING OTHER TECHNOLOGIES AS GENERALLY AVAILABLE IN PUBLICLY-FUNDED PRIMARY HEALTH-CARE FACILITIES

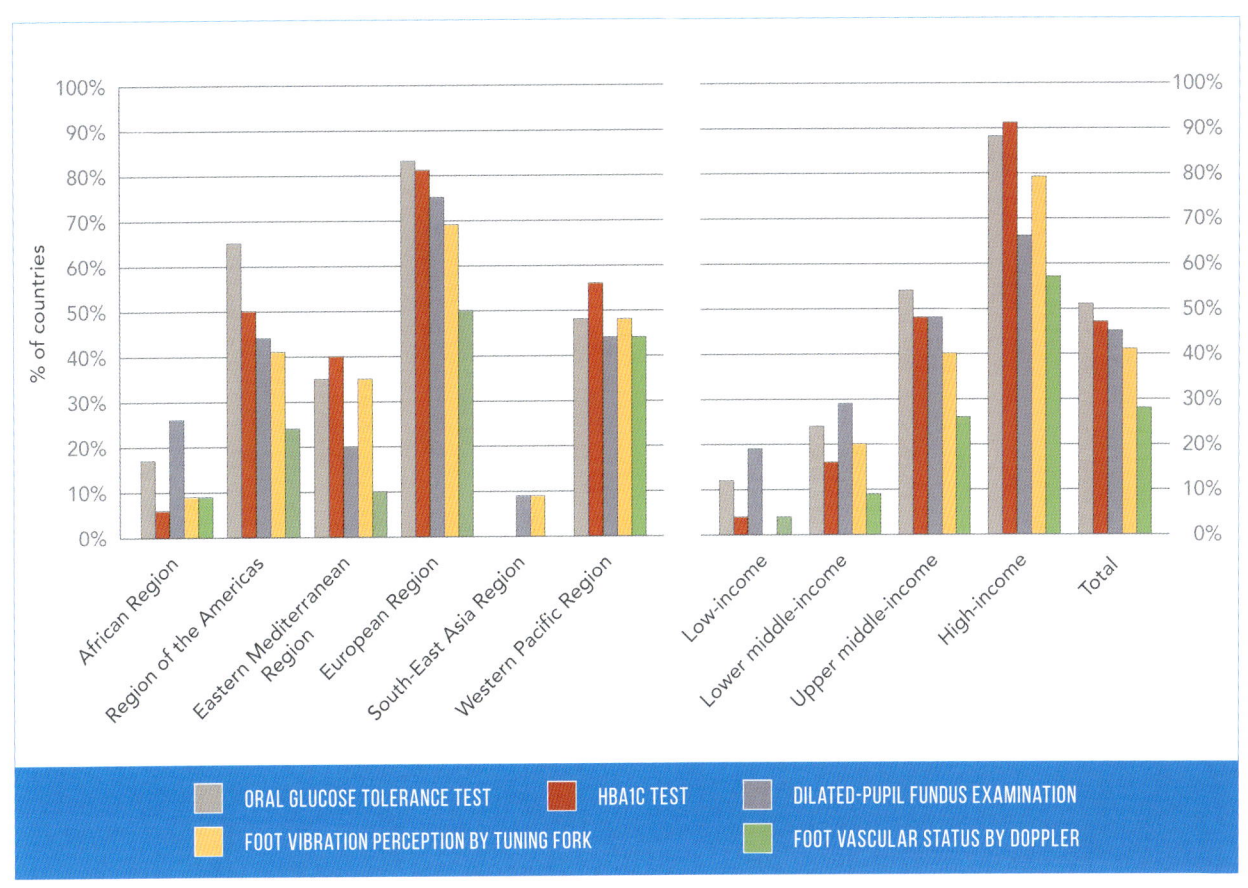

by dialysis, and 40% (71 countries) reported general availability of renal replacement by transplant. Among high-income countries, 93% (52 countries) report that renal replacement by dialysis is generally available, while in middle- and low-income countries it is 46% (47 countries) and 27% (seven countries) respectively.

4.4 SURVEILLANCE AND MONITORING

Regular population-based measurement of risk factors for type 2 diabetes is a key aspect of capacity to assess trends and impact of interventions. Less than 50% of countries reported conducting a national population-based survey with blood glucose measurement within the past 5 years. This low proportion partially reflects the cost and complexity associated with such measurement in surveys. WHO's Western Pacific Region had the highest achievement of surveys involving blood glucose measurement, with 80% of countries reporting one in the past 5 years. Countries in the WHO Eastern Mediterranean Region and the WHO European Region were least likely to have done a survey involving blood glucose measurement, with 25% and 27% of countries respectively reporting such a survey in the past 5 years.

Coverage of other risk factors was slightly better. Roughly two in three countries had conducted a national, population-based survey of overweight and obesity (72%) and physical inactivity (69%) in the past 5 years. Only 58% of countries conducted a national, population-based survey of overweight and obesity that involved measurement of height and weight.

Diabetes registries are specialized monitoring systems that can be a valuable resource to improve treatment compliance, prevent complications and assess the clinical outcomes of management. Globally, less than half of countries (44%) have a diabetes registry. Only 14% of countries reported having a registry which is population-based, whereas 19% reported a hospital-based registry, and 1% reported another kind of registry for diabetes. Low-income countries were least likely to have any kind of diabetes registry (19%) compared with middle- and high-income countries where it was 54% and 50% respectively.

4.5 SUMMARY

The results of the 2015 NCD CCS give an encouraging global impression that countries are taking action to address diabetes. Nearly three-quarters (72%) of countries have a national diabetes policy that is implemented with dedicated funding, and countries are also taking action at the policy level to address unhealthy diets and physical inactivity. Further efforts are needed to ensure funding and implementation of these policies and plans.

When it comes to setting standards to improve diabetes management, 71% of countries have national guidelines or standards, though less than half of countries are fully implementing them. Implementation of these standards can help to contain cost, optimize resources and ensure equitable service delivery, so mechanisms

Less than 50% of countries reported conducting a national population-based survey with blood glucose measurement

that kick-start locally appropriate implementation of national guidelines need to be explored. These might include periodic audits and the involvement of professional associations and patients' groups.

The availability of essential medicines and basic technologies in primary health care deserves further exploration, particularly in countries where basic technologies and essential medicines are not reported to be generally available.

Greater investment in data for surveillance and monitoring is called for, both through population-based surveys and incremental monitoring of diabetes *(4)*.

Finally, the NCD CCS findings presented in this chapter speak loudly that progress towards diabetes prevention and management is grossly uneven. HbA1c tests, considered the optimal tool for monitoring blood glucose levels (see Part 3), are mostly unavailable in low- and middle-income countries, but in many settings even more basic technologies for diagnosis and monitoring are also lacking. Among low- and lower middle-income countries, only one in three (35% and 36% of countries respectively) can report that the most basic technologies to measure height and weight, blood glucose, and urine strips for glucose and ketone measurement are generally available in primary care facilities. Insulin, along with metformin and sulphonylurea(s), is generally available in only a minority of low-income countries. This lack of access to basic technologies and essential medicines stands in sharp contrast to the reported widespread availability of these items in high-income countries.

Only 1 in 3 countries in lower income groups report general availability of the most basic technologies for diagnosis and management

REFERENCES

1. How WHO will report in 2017 to the United Nations General Assembly on the progress achieved in the implementation of commitments included in the 2011 UN Political Declaration and 2014 UN Outcome Document on NCDs (Technical note). Geneva: World Health Organization; 2015.

2. Noncommunicable diseases progress monitor 2015. Geneva: World Health Organization; 2015.

3. Implementation tools: Package of Essential Noncommunicable (PEN) Disease Interventions for Primary Health Care in Low-Resource Settings. Geneva: World Health Organization; 2013.

4. Global action plan for the prevention and control of noncommunicable diseases 2013–2020. Geneva: World Health Organization; 2013.

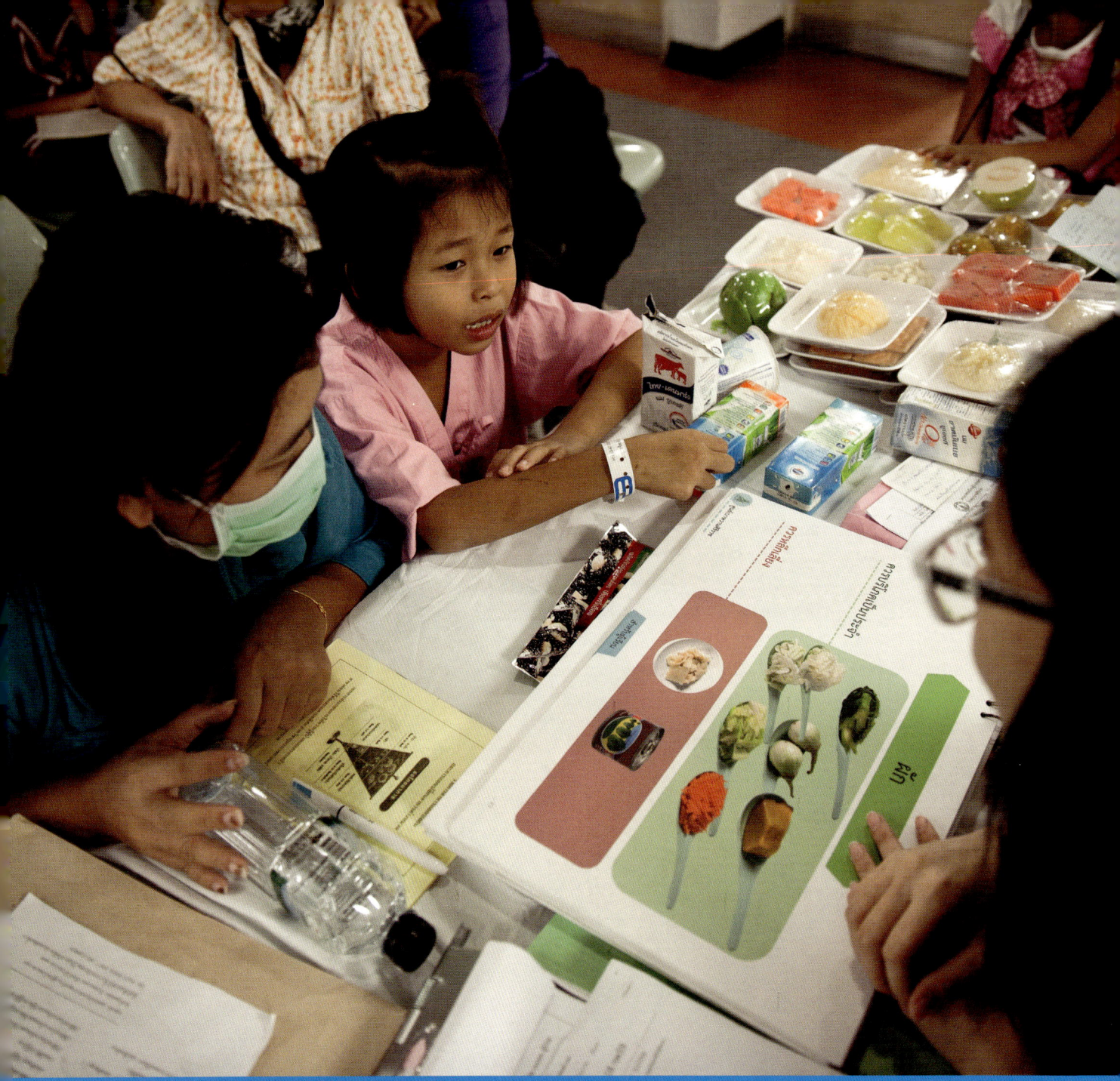

CONCLUSIONS AND RECOMMENDATIONS

SCALING-UP PREVENTION AND CONTROL OF DIABETES WITHIN AN INTEGRATED NCD RESPONSE

As the prevalence and numbers of people with diabetes continue to rise – a result of changes in the way people eat, move and live, and an ageing global population – the already-large health and economic impacts of diabetes will grow.

These impacts can be reduced through effective actions. With sufficient lifelong management and regular follow-up, people with all types of diabetes can live longer and healthier lives. The occurrence of type 2 diabetes can be reduced through population-based and individual prevention measures that target key risk factors.

Tackling diabetes is integral to the success of the overall response to NCDs. In most countries, commitments made through the Sustainable Development Goals – to reduce premature NCD mortality by a third by 2030, and to achieve universal health coverage – will require focused attention on diabetes prevention and management.

The data presented in this report indicate that many countries have begun to take action, evidenced by the high proportion of countries reporting national policies and plans related to diabetes prevention and control. Implementation, however, lags behind. Access to essential medicines and technologies appears to be a key obstacle to diabetes management, particularly in low- and middle-income countries. In many countries, lack of access to affordable insulin remains a key impediment to successful treatment and results in needless complications and premature deaths.

Guidance for effective diabetes prevention and control is set out in the *WHO Global action plan for the prevention and control of NCDs 2013–2020 (WHO NCD Global Action Plan)*, and a roadmap of national commitments to address diabetes is visible in the 2011 UN Political Declaration on NCDs and the 2014 UN Outcome Document on NCDs. The WHO NCD Global Action Plan global monitoring framework includes targets for 2025 to reduce mortality from diabetes and other NCDs, and a specific target to halt the rise in diabetes and obesity. In the context of an overall integrated approach to NCDs, Countries can take a series of actions, in line with the objectives of the WHO NCD Global Action Plan, to reduce the impact of diabetes:

1. ACCORD GREATER PRIORITY TO NCD PREVENTION AND CONTROL, INCLUDING DIABETES

Addressing NCDs, including diabetes, is an acknowledged priority for social development and investment in people. Scaling-up action for diabetes prevention and management with a wider NCD response requires high-level political commitment, resources, and effective leadership and advocacy – both national and international. Recommended actions for Member States to raise the priority of diabetes and NCDs include the following steps.

- Continue commitment to addressing diabetes as a priority in national NCD responses.

- Raise awareness about the national public health burden caused by diabetes and the relationship between diabetes, poverty and socioeconomic development.

- Consider establishing a national, multisectoral and high-level commission, agency or task force for engagement, policy coherence and mutual accountability among different spheres of policy-making that have a bearing on NCDs, in order to implement whole-of-government and whole-of-society approaches.

- Increase and prioritize national budgetary allocations for addressing diabetes and key risk factors.

2. STRENGTHEN NATIONAL CAPACITY TO ACCELERATE COUNTRY RESPONSE

The lead responsibility for ensuring appropriate legislative, regulatory, financial and service arrangements for diabetes prevention and management lies with government. Integrated, multisectoral action and accountability are necessary for success. In the context of existing commitments to address NCD prevention and management, recommended actions to strengthen national capacity to address diabetes include the following steps.

- Strengthen the capacity of ministries of health to exercise a strategic leadership and coordination role in policy development that engages all stakeholders across government, nongovernmental organizations, civil society and the private sector, ensuring that issues relating to diabetes receive a coordinated, comprehensive and integrated response.

- Ensure that national policies and plans addressing diabetes are fully costed and then funded and implemented. Make use of all available data on exposure to the known risk factors for type 2 diabetes, diabetes prevalence and the complications of diabetes to inform provisions in the national plan for diabetes prevention and management.

- Foster accountability by setting national targets and indicators for diabetes, obesity, physical inactivity, availability of essential medicines and basic technologies, and reductions in premature mortality resulting from NCDs, taking into account the global NCD targets for 2025 and the NCD-related Sustainable Development Goal targets for 2030.

- Include interventions for the prevention and control of diabetes within existing national programmes for nutrition, physical activity and sport, maternal and child health, cardiovascular disease, and communicable diseases such as HIV/AIDS and tuberculosis, especially in primary care.

3. CREATE, SUSTAIN AND EXPAND HEALTH-PROMOTING ENVIRONMENTS TO REDUCE MODIFIABLE RISK FACTORS

The key modifiable risk factors for type 2 diabetes are overweight and obesity, insufficient physical activity and unhealthy dietary practices. Smoking also increases the risk of type 2 diabetes, as well as the risk of diabetes-related complications. Reducing these factors will decrease the occurrence of type 2 diabetes and reduce complications related to all types of diabetes. It will also lead to reductions in other NCDs such as cardiovascular disease.

Preventing people becoming overweight or obese is a priority for reducing type 2 diabetes. Many of the risks start in the womb, and nutrition and health during the antenatal period are critical. Promotion of breastfeeding, and healthier diet and physical activity in childhood and adolescence along with other supportive environments, can contribute to healthier people and reduction in diabetes and NCDs.

Culturally and environmentally appropriate strategies are needed to create environments that support people to maintain healthy body weight, healthy diet, and physical activity. Recommended actions include the following steps.

- Promote the intake of healthy foods and reduce the intake of unhealthy food and sugar-sweetened beverages. Policy tools include fiscal measures to raise the price of sugar-sweetened beverages and unhealthy foods and/or lower the price of healthier foods; regulation of marketing of food and non-alcoholic beverages to children; nutrition labelling; and a package of interventions to improve early childhood nutrition, including promotion of breastfeeding.

- Create supportive built and social environments for physical activity – transport and urban planning policy measures can facilitate access to safe, affordable opportunities for physical activity. Point-of-decision prompts can encourage more active transport – to use stairs versus a lift, for example.

- Maximize impact with multicomponent programmes involving policy changes, settings-based interventions, mass media campaigns and education. Prioritize highly vulnerable and/or disadvantaged groups.

In addition to measures to promote healthy diet and physical activity, reducing exposure to tobacco will reduce the complications of diabetes and may lead to reductions in type 2 diabetes. Tobacco use can be reduced through implementation of comprehensive tobacco control measures in line with WHO's Framework Convention on Tobacco Control.

4. STRENGTHEN AND ORIENT HEALTH SYSTEMS TO ADDRESS DIABETES

Improvements in diabetes management will reduce rates of complications, ease pressure on health systems and improve quality of life for people living with diabetes.

The core components of diabetes management include diagnosis; health education and counselling to promote healthy choices and self-care; medications in some cases; screening and treatment of complications; and consistent follow-up. Provision of these building blocks of care in a primary health-care setting requires adequate health infrastructure and planning.

Diabetes management should be part of national NCD management and be incorporated into the package of essential services included in universal health coverage. Recommended actions to strengthen diabetes management include the following steps.

- Adapt and implement a primary health-care package for the diagnosis and effective management of all types of diabetes, including management protocols and referral criteria, in the context of integrated NCD management.

- Implement policies and programmes to ensure equitable access to affordable essential medicines (including life-saving insulin) and technologies (including diagnostic equipment and supplies).

- Enhance the skills and capacity of health-care providers to provide comprehensive care for diabetes.

- Promote education and awareness around self-care practices and regular check-ups to facilitate early detection and treatment of complications.

5. PROMOTE HIGH-QUALITY RESEARCH AND DEVELOPMENT

There is evidence for effective interventions to improve management of diabetes and to reduce its modifiable risk factors, but there are significant gaps in the knowledge base. WHO's prioritized research agenda for prevention and control of NCDs outlines key areas of diabetes-related research. Recommended research to advance diabetes prevention and control includes the following areas.

- Ongoing research into risk factors and prevention of all types of diabetes.

- Innovative intervention research to expand the evidence base for promotion of physical activity.

- Innovative outcome evaluation to capture the impact of environmental change on overweight and obesity, and on type 2 diabetes.

- Implementation research to better understand the scope and scale of health-system strengthening.

- Options to improve access to insulin.

6. MONITOR TRENDS AND DETERMINANTS, AND EVALUATE PROGRESS

Monitoring progress in diabetes prevention and control requires establishing and strengthening appropriate surveillance mechanisms, as well as the capacity to make use of the resulting data. Recommended actions for strengthening diabetes surveillance and monitoring include the following steps.

- Introduce or strengthen existing vital registration and cause of death registration systems to better reflect the role of diabetes as the primary or underlying cause of death.

- Strengthen national capacity to collect, analyse and use representative data on the diabetes burden and trends.

- Conduct periodic population-level surveys that include measurement of risk factors and blood glucose. Use information from risk factor surveys and country capacity surveys, and modify plans and programmes as necessary.

- Develop, maintain and strengthen a diabetes registry if feasible and sustainable, and include information on complications. This can be more easily achieved when electronic medical files are used.

This first *WHO Global report on diabetes* underscores the enormous size of the problem, and also the potential to reverse current trends. The political basis for concerted action to address diabetes is there, woven into the Sustainable Development Goals, the United Nations Political Declaration on NCDs, and the WHO NCD Global Action Plan 2013–2020. Where built upon, these foundations will catalyse action by all.

There are no simple solutions for addressing diabetes but coordinated, multicomponent intervention can make a significant difference. Everyone has a role to play – governments, health-care providers, people with diabetes and those who care for them, civil society, food producers, and manufacturers and suppliers of medicines and technology are all stakeholders. Collectively, they can all make a significant contribution to halt the rise in diabetes and improve the lives of those living with the disease.

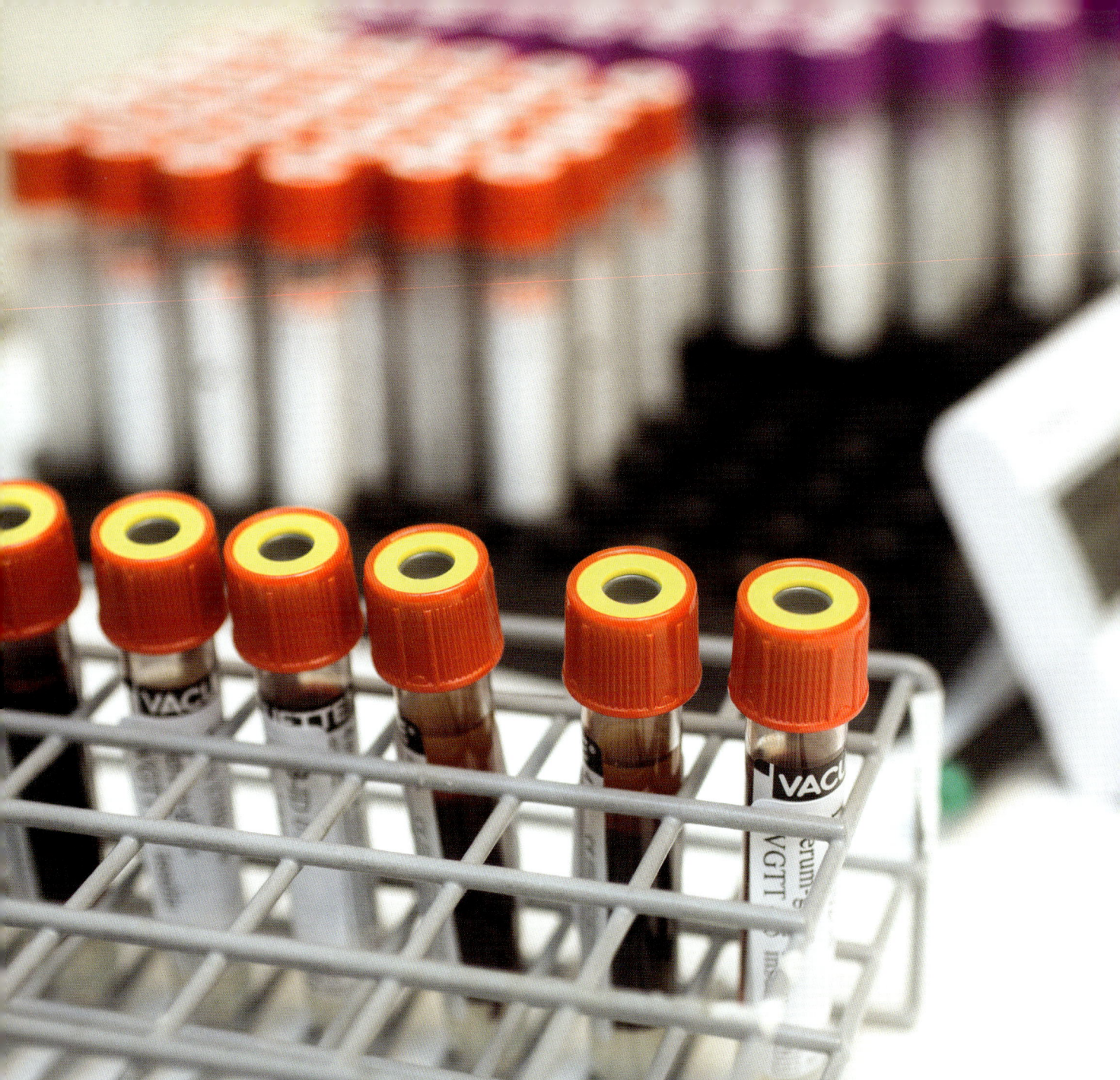

ANNEXES

ANNEX A. CURRENT WHO RECOMMENDATIONS FOR THE DIAGNOSTIC CRITERIA FOR DIABETES AND INTERMEDIATE HYPERGLYCAEMIA

Diabetes	
Fasting plasma glucose	≥7.0 mmol/L (126 mg/dl)
	or
2-h plasma glucose*	≥11.1 mmol/L (200 mg/dl)
	or
HbA1c	≥6.5%
Impaired glucose tolerance (IGT)	
Fasting plasma glucose	<7.0 mmol/L (126 mg/dl)
	and
2-h plasma glucose*	≥7.8 and <11.1 mmol/L (140 mg/dl and 200 mg/dl)
Impaired fasting glucose (IFG)	
Fasting plasma glucose	6.1 to 6.9 mmol/L (110 mg/dl to 125 mg/dl)
	and (if measured)
2-h plasma glucose*	<7.8 mmol/L (140 mg/dl)
Gestational diabetes (GDM)	
One or more of the following:	
Fasting plasma glucose	5.1–6.9 mmol/L (92–125 mgl/dl)
1-h plasma glucose**	≥10.0 mmol/L (180 mg/dl)
2-h plasma glucose	8.5–11.0 mmol/L (153–199 mg/dl)

* Venous plasma glucose 2 hours after ingestion of 75 g oral glucose load
** Venous plasma glucose 1 hour after ingestion of 75 g oral glucose load

In people who do not have symptoms, a positive test for diabetes should be repeated on another day.[1]
Blood glucose measurement is relatively simple and cheap and should be available at primary health-care level.

---

1. *Source: Definition and diagnosis of diabetes and intermediate hyperglycaemia. Geneva: World Health Organization; 2006.*

ANNEX B. METHODS FOR ESTIMATING DIABETES PREVALENCE, OVERWEIGHT AND OBESITY PREVALENCE, MORTALITY ATTRIBUTABLE TO HIGH BLOOD GLUCOSE, AND PRICE OF INSULIN

Data in this report were derived from a number of sources, each of which is explained below. They are not necessarily the official statistics of Member States.

PREVALENCE OF DIABETES AND TRENDS IN MEAN FASTING PLASMA GLUCOSE LEVELS

The diabetes prevalence data presented in this report were estimated by the NCD Risk Factor Collaboration (NCD-RisC) – a worldwide network/consortium of public health and medical researchers and practitioners who together work with the World Health Organization to document NCD risk factors and their health effects around the world. Diabetes prevalence and mean fasting plasma glucose (FPG) were estimated in the adult population (18 years and older) for the years 1980 and 2014. Diabetes was defined as fasting plasma glucose levels >=7.0 mmol/L (126 mg/dl); or using insulin or oral hypoglycaemic drugs; or having a history of diagnosis of diabetes *(1)*.

To estimate diabetes prevalence and mean fasting plasma glucose by country for the years 1980 and 2014, NCD-RisC used data provided to WHO or to the NCD-RisC group *(1)*. Inclusion criteria for analysis were that the data had come from a random sample of a national, subnational, or community population, with clearly described survey methods and a clearly specified definition of diabetes, and which had measured one of the following biomarkers: FPG, 2-hour oral glucose tolerance test (2hOGTT), and/or HbA1c. Regressions were used to convert any prevalence data that had been defined using alternative definitions of diabetes, such as definitions using 2hOGTT and FPG, or based on an alternative FPG cut-off. Statistical models were used to estimate prevalence and mean fasting plasma glucose by country and year (for description, see *(2)* in references). Uncertainty in estimates was analysed by taking into account sampling error and uncertainty due to statistical modelling. For comparison by regional groupings and time trends, prevalence estimates were age-adjusted using the Standard WHO Population *(3)*.

The estimates are an update of estimates for the same year published in the Global status report on NCDs 2014 *(4)*, as they include additional survey data.

PREVALENCE OF OVERWEIGHT AND OBESITY

The prevalence of overweight and obesity data presented in this report were estimated by NCD-RisC, in the adult population (18 years and older) for 2014 *(5)*. Overweight was defined as the percentage of the population aged 18 or older having a body mass index (BMI) ≥25 kg/m2. Obesity was defined as the percentage of the population aged 18 or older having a body mass index (BMI) ≥30 kg/m2. NCD-RisC used data provided to WHO or to the NCD-RisC group. Inclusion criteria for analysis were that the data had come from a random sample of a national, subnational, or community population, with clearly described survey methods and with height and weight measured in the study population. Statistical models were used to estimate prevalence by country and year (for description, see *(5)* in references). Uncertainty in estimates was analysed by taking into account sampling error and uncertainty due to statistical modelling. For comparison by regional groupings and time trends, prevalence estimates were age-adjusted using the Standard WHO Population *(3)*.

MORTALITY ATTRIBUTABLE TO DIABETES AND HIGH BLOOD GLUCOSE

Age and sex-specific, all-cause mortality rates were estimated for 2000–2012 from revised life tables published in World Health Statistics 2014 *(6)*. Detailed information on the methodology is available in WHO methods and data sources for country-level causes of death 2000–2012 *(7)*. The total number of deaths by age and sex was estimated for each country by applying these death rates to the estimated population prepared by the United Nations Population Division in its 2012 revision *(8)*. Causes of death were estimated for 2000–2012 using data sources and methods described by WHO in 2014 *(9)*. Vital registration systems that record deaths with sufficient completeness were used as the preferred data source. The mortality estimates are based on a combination of country life tables, cause of death models and regional cause of death patterns.

There is convincing evidence for a causal relationship between higher-than-optimal fasting blood glucose levels and cardiovascular disease (CVD), chronic kidney disease, and tuberculosis (TB) mortality. The optimal distribution of fasting blood glucose is estimated to be population distribution with a mean of 4.9–5.3 mmol/L, SD 0.4–0.6, which are levels corresponding to lowest all-cause mortality as derived from meta-analyses of prospective studies *(10)*. Relative risks of higher-than-optimal fasting plasma glucose were derived from meta-analyses of prospective studies *(10, 11)*. Population-attributable fractions for each age-sex group and each country were calculated using the estimated distribution of FPG and relative risks for each cause of death (CVD, chronic kidney disease, and TB). The number of deaths attributable to high blood glucose was calculated by multiplying the population-attributable fraction for CVD deaths, chronic kidney disease deaths and TB deaths by the number of deaths from each cause for each age-sex-country unit. All deaths with diabetes assigned as the underlying cause of death are assumed to be caused by higher-than-optimal blood glucose. More details on the methodology are available elsewhere *(12)*.

ASSESSING NATIONAL RESPONSE TO DIABETES PREVENTION AND CONTROL

Assessment of national capacity indicators related to diabetes prevention management was based on Member State responses to the 2015 Noncommunicable Disease Country Capacity Survey (NCD CCS) *(13)*.

The NCD CCS is conducted periodically by WHO to assess individual country capacity for NCD prevention. A first survey was conducted in 2000, followed by surveys in 2005, 2010, 2013 and 2015. The questionnaire covers health system infrastructure; funding; policies, plans and strategies; surveillance; primary health care; and partnerships and multilateral collaboration. The 2015 NCD CCS was completed by national NCD focal points or designated colleagues within the ministry of health or a national institute/agency. The questions were designed to obtain objective information about the adequacy of capacity, and countries were requested to provide supporting documentation to enable review by WHO in order to validate the responses. Where discrepancies were noted between the country response and the provided supporting documents or other available sources of information at WHO, clarification was requested from the countries. The 2015 NCD CCS was completed through a web-based platform between May and August 2015. Of 194 Member States, 177 responded to the survey, representing 97% of the world's population. More information on the NCD CCS, including the questionnaire and past survey reports, is available on the survey website (*http://www.who.int/chp/ncd_capacity/en/*).

PRICE OF INSULIN

Management Sciences for Health (MSH) is a non-profit organisation established in 1971 *(14)*. Since its establishment it has worked in over 150 countries to develop health systems, focusing on improving quality, availability and affordability of health services. One of the tools developed by MSH is the International Drug Price Indicator Guide (IDPIG) *(15)*. The guide provides a variety of prices from different sources including pharmaceutical suppliers, international development agencies and governments. This guide allows for comparison of prices of medicines of assured quality and is used as a reference in many approaches looking at access to medicines, for example the methodology developed by WHO and Health Action International *(16)*.

Using the online version of IDPIG, data from 1996 to 2014 were extracted from purchasers of insulin. All insulin formulations were standardized to an equivalent of a 10 ml 100 IU vial. The minimum, maximum and median prices are calculated over the time period for all countries combined, as well as median prices over the time period, disaggregated by country income group as defined by the World Bank in 2015.

REFERENCES

1. NCD Risk Factor Collaboration (NCD-RisC). Worldwide trends in diabetes since 1980: a pooled analysis of 751 population-based studies with 4*4 million participants. Lancet 2016; published online April 7. http://dx.doi.org/10.1016/S0140-6736(16)00618-8.

2. Finucane MM, Danaei G, Ezzati M. Bayesian estimation of population-level trends in measures of health status. Statistical Sciences. 2014;29;18–25.

3. Ahmad O. Age standardization of rates: a new WHO standard (Technical report). GPE discussion paper series: No 31. Geneva: World Health Organization; 2001.

4. Global status report on noncommunicable diseases 2014. Geneva: World Health Organization; 2014.

5. NCD Risk Factor Collaboration (NCD-RisC). Trends in adult body-mass index in 200 countries from 1975 to 2014: a pooled analysis of 1698 population-based measurement studies with 19*2 million participants. Lancet (in press).

6. World Health Statistics 2014. Geneva: World Health Organization; 2014.

7. WHO methods for life expectancy and healthy life expectancy. Global health estimates technical paper WHO/HIS/HSI/GHE/2014.5. Geneva: World Health Organization; 2014.

8. United Nations Population Division. World population prospects – 2012 revision. New York: United Nations; 2013.

9. WHO methods and data sources for country-level causes of death 2000–2012. Global health estimates technical paper WHO/HIS/HSI/GHE/2014.7. Geneva: World Health Organization; 2014.

10. Singh GM, Danaei G, Farzadfar F, Stevens GA, Woodward M, Wormser DK, et al. The age-specific quantitative effects of metabolic risk factors on cardiovascular diseases and diabetes: a pooled analysis. PLoS. One. 2013;8,:(7)e65174.

11. Jeon CY, Murray MB. Diabetes mellitus increases the risk of active tuberculosis: a systematic review of 13 observational studies. PLoS.Med. 2008;5:(7)e152.

12. Global Burden of Metabolic Risk Factors for Chronic Diseases Collaboration. Cardiovascular disease, chronic kidney disease and diabetes mortality burden of cardiometabolic risk factors from 1980 to 2010: a comparative risk assessment. Lancet Diabetes Endocrinology. 2014;2:(8)634–647.

13. Noncommunicable diseases progress monitor, 2015. Geneva: World Health Organization; 2015.

14. Mission and Vision. Medford, Massachusettes: Management Sciences for Health; 2015.

15. International Drug Price Indicator Guide, 2015. Washington DC: Management Sciences for Health; 2015.

16. Measuring medicine prices, availability, affordability and price components Geneva and Amsterdam: World Health Organization and Health Action International; 2008.